Elena Hernández-Jiménez

CHEMICAL PEELING

IN COSMETIC DERMATOLOGY & SKINCARE PRACTICE

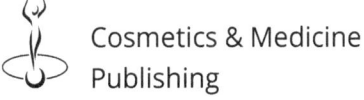
Cosmetics & Medicine Publishing

Author:
Elena I. Hernández-Jiménez, *Ph.D.*

CHEMICAL PEELING
IN COSMETIC DERMATOLOGY AND SKINCARE PRACTICE

Chemical peeling (chemoexfoliation) has been one of the most popular skincare and cosmetic dermatology treatments for many years. Its popularity is well deserved because it makes it possible to solve different aesthetic problems effectively and with minimal risks. Yes, this is true, but with one caveat: if the peeling is done correctly. "Correctly" means not only the procedure itself. The peel product, skin pre-treatment, and following restorative care must be chosen and performed by a qualified professional in line with the patient's needs and health status. There are many nuances, and the specialist's skill is to take them all into account.

This book presents all the most important facts you should know and remember when working with chemoexfoliation — from the chemical nature of different peeling agents and their effects on skin cells to the clinical effect, from indications and contraindications to the features of the procedure. The book reflects up-to-date knowledge and views about the purposes, mechanisms of action, and clinical possibilities of chemical peeling with a proven basis.

The book consists of four parts. The first part reveals the essence of the method named "chemical peeling" and discusses its clinical capabilities and limitations in general.

The second part describes different types of chemical peels — keratolytic, acid, enzymatic, and retinol. Although there are some similarities in the main clinical outcomes (skin scaling), the peeling agents differ in their chemical nature, targets in the skin, and mechanisms. In addition to general indications and contraindications, each chemical peeling type has peculiarities in the procedure, and our book explains why this is so.

The third part presents a discussion on the general principles of chemical peeling — the choice of the peel formulation, the skin preparation for the procedure, the procedure itself, and the subsequent rehabilitation. There is also information about the influence of nutrition on the clinical results of chemical peeling.

The fourth part focuses on the usefulness of instrumental assessment of skin conditions before and after the chemical peeling. Objective data on the initial state of the barrier function of the patient's skin helps the practitioner to select the optimal peel product, determine the interval between the procedures, and monitor the skin's recovery. This reduces the risks of unwanted reactions and achieves the best possible clinical results.

ISBN 978-1-970196-27-6 (paperback)
ISBN 978-1-970196-37-5 (hardcover)
ISBN 978-1-970196-02-3 (eBook — Adobe PDF)
ISBN 978-1-970196-26-9 (eBook — ePUB)

© Cosmetics & Medicine Publishing LLC, 2024
© Cover photo: Blackday / Shutterstock

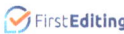

English version is edited and certified by the FirstEditing.Com, Inc. (USA).

Author/Editor

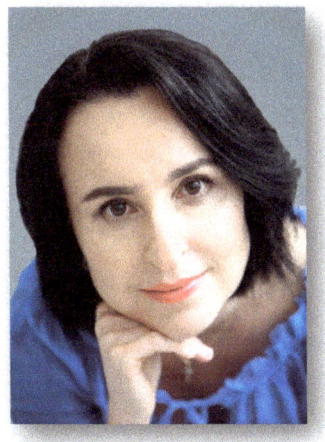

Elena I. Hernández-Jiménez, *Ph.D.*

Biophysicist, scientific journalist

Editor-in-chief of Cosmetics and Medicine Publishing

Chairperson of the Executive Board of the International Society of Applied Corneotherapy (I.A.C.)

Author and co-author of numerous publications in professional magazines, co-author and editor of the book series *Fundamentals of Cosmetic Dermatology & Skincare, Cosmetic Dermatology & Skincare Practice, Cosmetic Chemistry for Dermatology & Skincare Specialists* and others

Speaker at international conferences, author of training seminars and webinars for professionals in the field of skincare

Professional interests: biology and physiology of the skin, skin permeability, cosmetic chemistry, anti-age medicine, physiotherapy in dermatology and aesthetic medicine, skin analysis and imaging

Table of Contents

Abbreviations 9
Introduction 10

PART I
CHEMICAL PEELING: THE ESSENCE OF THE TREATMENT

1.1. Clinical effects 13
    1.1.1. General indications for chemical peeling:
          epidermal problems 14
    1.1.2. General contraindications 16
1.2. Biological basis 16
    1.2.1. Chemical peeling is based on the skin's ability
          to renew itself 16
    1.2.2. Epidermis, the primary target for chemical peels 17
    1.2.3. Chemical peeling "inside-out" and "outside-in":
          what's the difference? 19

PART II
TYPES OF CHEMICAL PEELS

Chapter 1. Keratolytic peels 22
1.1. Features of keratolytic peels 22
    1.1.1. Mechanism of action 22
    1.1.2. Skin targets for keratolytic agents 23
          Skin surface 23
          Living layers 24
    1.1.3. Features of keratolytic peeling 25
1.2. Trichloroacetic acid 27
    1.2.1. Mechanism of action 27
    1.2.2. Safety aspects 29
    1.2.3. Practical aspects 30

1.2.4. Modified TCA for chemical skin remodeling 32
1.3. Phenol... 34
    1.3.1. Mechanism of action 35
    1.3.2. Safety aspects.. 36
    1.3.3. Practical aspects... 40
1.4. Salicylic acid and lipohydroxy acid (LHA) 41
    1.4.1. Mechanism of action and clinical effects 43
    1.4.2. Indications and contraindications 44
    1.4.3. Practical aspects... 46
1.5. Resorcinol and Jessner peel....................................... 46
    1.5.1. Mechanism of action 47
    1.5.2. Safety aspects.. 47
    1.5.3. Modified Jessner peel 48

Chapter 2. Acid peels 49
2.1. Hydroxy acids: chemical structure and classification 50
2.2. Mechanism of action 51
2.3. α-Hydroxy acids (AHAs)... 56
    2.3.1. AHAs for topical application 56
        Glycolic acid.. 56
        Lactic acid 57
        Pyruvic acid 58
        Mandelic acid 59
        Tartaric acid... 59
        Malic acid.. 60
        Citric acid.. 60
    2.3.2. Clinical effects 61
        Scaling... 61
        Moisturizing... 61
        Soothing... 62
    2.3.3. Features of AHA-containing formulations 62
        Combinations of active ingredients............................ 63
        Optimal base.. 64
        pH of the finished product 65

2.3.4. Indications and practical aspects 65
    Skincare routine, age-related changes prevention,
    and treatment 65
    Acne, post-acne 67
    Atopic dermatitis 68
    Pseudofolliculitis barbae 68
    Ichthyosis 69
    Keratosis 69
    Warts 71
2.3.5. Contraindications and safety 71
2.4. Polyhydroxy acids (PHAs) 73
  2.4.1. Lactobionic acid 73
  2.4.2. Gluconic acid and gluconolactone 74

Chapter 3. Enzymatic peels 77
3.1. *Stratum corneum*'s proteases: types and functions 78
  3.1.1. Proteases and antiproteases 79
    Serine proteases 80
    Aspartate proteases 81
    Cysteine proteases 81
    Antiproteases 82
  3.1.2. Aesthetic treatments affecting the *stratum corneum*'s
       protease activity 83
3.2. Prescription features of enzymatic peels 85
  3.2.1. Proteases — the main active components
       of enzymatic peels 85
    Plant proteases 85
    Proteases of microbial origin 87
    Proteases of animal origin 87
    Modified natural peptidases 88
  3.2.2. How to keep the enzyme active 89
  3.2.3. Combining enzymes with other peeling agents
       in one formulation 90
    Enzymes + salicylic acid 90
    Enzymes + AHAs 92

3.3. Clinical effects 93
3.4. Practical aspects 95
    3.4.1. Indications and contraindications 95
    3.4.2. How to perform enzymatic peeling 98
    3.4.3. How enzymatic exfoliants are combined
          with AHA-based peels 99

Chapter 4. Retinol peels 101
4.1. Retinol and its derivatives: structure, metabolism,
    mechanism of action 101
    4.1.1. Retinol — the first in the series of vitamins 101
    4.1.2. Retinol transformations in the body and the cell 103
    4.1.3. Synthetic retinoids 108
    4.1.4. Plant retinoids 109
    4.1.5. How to explain the variety of clinical effects
          of retinoids 110
4.2. Dermal effects of retinoids 111
    4.2.1. Keratinocytes and keratinization of the epidermis 114
    4.2.2. Sebocytes and acne 115
    4.2.3. Hair follicle cells and hair loss 116
    4.2.4. Langerhans cells and skin immunity 117
    4.2.5. Melanocytes and skin pigmentation 118
    4.2.6. Fibroblasts and wrinkle smoothing 119
4.3. Topical retinoids in cosmetic dermatology and skincare 120
    4.3.1. Drugs and cosmetic formulations 121
    4.3.2. Adverse effects and contraindications
          to the use of retinol cosmetics 122
4.4. Prescription features of retinol products 123
    4.4.1. Choosing the optimal dose 123
    4.4.2. How to keep retinol active 124
    4.4.3. Combination with other active substances 126
4.5. Peculiarities of retinol peeling "within-out" 127
4.6. Practical aspects 128

PART III
GENERAL PRINCIPLES OF CHEMICAL PEELING

1.1. Choice of peel formulation 132
1.2. Pre-peeling 136
1.3. Peeling procedure 138
    1.3.1. Skin cleansing 138
    1.3.2. During the procedure 139
1.4. Post-treatment rehabilitation 140
    1.4.1. Calming agents and inflammation 141
    1.4.2. Occlusive agents and barrier function 143
    1.4.3. UV filters and sun protection 143
1.5. Influence of nutrition on the clinical effect of chemical peeling 145
    1.5.1. Pre-peeling preparation 145
    1.5.2. Rehabilitation 146

PART IV
INSTRUMENTAL ASSESSMENT OF SKIN CONDITION AND AFTER-PEELING SUPPORT OF BARRIER FUNCTION

1.1. Symptoms of skin damage after chemical peeling 148
1.2. Post-peeling dryness: causes, assessment, treatment 150
    1.2.1. Desquamation 153
    1.2.2. Transepidermal water loss 154
    1.2.3. Sebum 155
    1.2.4. Hydration 158
1.3. Comprehensive approach to the assessment and treatment of dryness 159

References 161

Abbreviations

AHA	—	alpha hydroxy acid
BHA	—	beta hydroxy acid
CGRP	—	calcitonin gene-related peptide
CRABP	—	cellular retinoic acid-binding protein
CRBP	—	cellular retinol-binding protein
CROSS	—	chemical reconstruction of skin scars
DNA	—	deoxyribonucleic acid
EDTA	—	ethylenediaminetetraacetic acid
FDA	—	U.S. Food and Drug Administration
IL	—	interleukin
IPL	—	intense pulse light
LHA	—	lipohydroxy acid
LLLT	—	low-level laser therapy
NADH	—	nicotinamide adenine dinucleotide
NMF	—	natural moisturizing factor
pH	—	*pondus Hydrogenii* (hydrogen index)
PHA	—	polyhydroxy acid
PRP	—	platelet-rich plasma
RA	—	retinoic acid
RAR	—	retinoic acid receptor
RF	—	radio frequency
RNA	—	ribonucleic acid
ROS	—	reactive oxygen species
RXR	—	retinoid X receptor
SP	—	substance P
SPF	—	sun protection factor
TCA	—	trichloroacetic acid
TCAA	—	trichloroacetate ammonium
TEWL	—	transepidermal water loss
US	—	ultrasound
UV	—	ultraviolet
UVA	—	ultraviolet type A
UVB	—	ultraviolet type B

Introduction

For many years, chemical peeling has remained one of the most popular methods in skincare and cosmetic dermatology. This prominent status is well deserved because it helps solve many aesthetic and dermatological problems effectively and with minimal risks.

Yes, this is true, but with one proviso: **the chemical peeling must be done correctly**. "Correctly" means not only the procedure but also the choice of the peel formulation, skin preparation for the chemical treatment, and special rehabilitation after the procedure must be optimal for the given patient. To achieve these aims, there are many practical nuances the professional must consider.

In the *Chemical Peeling in Cosmetic Dermatology & Skincare Practice* book, we have collected all the most important details those working with chemical peels need to know and remember when working with chemical peels.

- What chemical peels are there, and how do they differ?
- What aesthetic problems can (and cannot) be solved by chemical peeling?
- How will the peeling agent behave in contact with the skin?
- What are the targets, and how do the peeling agents affect them?
- How will the skin react to the procedure and why?
- What criteria must a chemical peel formulation meet?
- What effects can be expected from each chemical peel type?
- What are the indications and contraindications for their use and why?
- How to choose a chemical peel and adequately perform the procedure?

These and many other practical questions are discussed in detail in our book based on the available evidence. Although it is primarily intended for practitioners — beauticians, skincare specialists, and dermatologists — it is of interest to anyone who cares about their health and wants to understand the possibilities of modern skincare and cosmetic dermatology.

Part I

Chemical peeling: the essence of the treatment

1.1. Clinical effects

The skin undergoes structural changes that negatively affect its appearance and functions due to aging, external (e.g., ultraviolet/UV radiation, pollution, extremely cold/hot temperatures), and internal (e.g., diseases, psycho-emotional stress, imbalanced nutrition) aggressors. These changes are observed in all skin layers, including the epidermis and the main skin barrier — the *stratum corneum*. Of all the methods available today in cosmetic and aesthetic dermatology influencing the *stratum corneum*, the most effective is the use of topical formulations capable of stimulating and accelerating the epidermal cell renewal (proliferation, migration, and differentiation of keratinocytes) and the formation of the *stratum corneum* barrier structures (keratinization and desquamation).

These formulations are combined into a group of peel products.

Definitions

Peeling is a general name for methods (chemical, physical, mechanical) exfoliating (partially or entirely) the *stratum corneum*, as well as affecting the underlying layers of the epidermis, to initiate skin regeneration processes.

Chemical peeling (or **chemoexfoliation**) is performed by applying particular substances (so-called **peeling agents**) to cause controlled skin damage through chemical reactions between skin components and the agent. Topical formulations for chemical peeling, having in their composition peeling agents, are called **peel products** (or **chemical peels**).

The result of peeling is active **skin scaling** induced by massive "shedding" of corneocytes which signals to the basal keratinocytes to accelerate their division to restore the skin barrier structures as quickly as possible.

Chemical peeling is probably the most ancient way to "renew" the skin: information about the magic effect of fruit pulp or fermented milk can be found in old manuscripts and folk tales. For example, keratolytic formulas were discussed in a famous ancient Egyptian medical papyrus (dated 1352 B.C., found and published in 1875 by the German Egyptologist Georg Ebers). It also described cosmetic scrub: the Egyptians used a mixture of alabaster particles with honey and milk to cleanse and care for the skin.

The era of chemical peels began with the work of the German dermatologist Paul Gerson Unna. In 1882 Unna published the methodology and results of such exfoliating agents as trichloroacetic acid (TCA), salicylic acid, phenol, and resorcinol. Thanks to these works, we know that German dermatologists already used these substances and their combinations in the 19th century to correct acne scars, brighten age spots, and relieve ichthyosis symptoms. The main problem was the toxicity of the ingredients used: phenol and TCA penetrate the skin quickly, and the amount released into the blood could be fatal if treatment is performed over a large body area. Therefore, physicians used phenol peels only when necessary to correct demoralizing aesthetic imperfections.

Since then, the choice of peel products has significantly expanded. Today, a wide range of products based on salicylic acid, fruit acids, proteolytic enzymes, and retinol are available on the market. With the advent of safer products and the development of injection and physical technologies that allow safe "work" in deep skin layers, phenol and TCA have left the legal cosmetics market because of high toxicity, traumatism, and difficulty of control during the procedure.

1.1.1. General indications for chemical peeling: epidermal problems

Currently, chemical peeling is used to solve aesthetic problems of **epidermal origin**, i.e., those that appeared due to changes in the epidermis.

Epidermal problems can be divided into two main groups:
1. **Textural changes related to impaired keratinization** — surface wrinkles, roughness
2. **Color changes associated with impaired pigment formation and lipofuscin accumulation in cells** — dyschromia (hypo- or hyper-pigmentation, dullness, tint — yellowish, reddish, grayish)

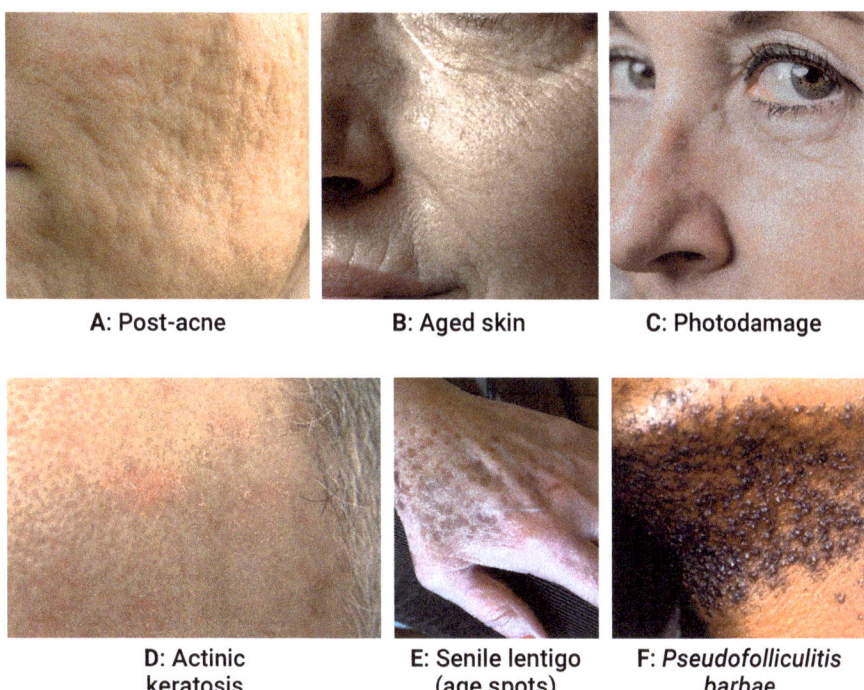

Figure I-1. General indications for chemical peeing (Images by: A–C — Freepik.com, D–F — Wikipedia.com)

In the pathogenesis and clinical picture of many skin conditions or even pathologies, there are often several epidermal problems at once (**Fig. I-1**), which is the reason for the use of chemical peels.

For example, with **post-acne**, pigmentation disorders and altered topography are observed. Keratosis, uneven tone, and superficial wrinkles are the components of **aging skin syndrome**. Pigmentation disorders and coarsening are characteristic of **photodamaged skin**. Pathologies such as actinic keratosis, age spots (senile lentigo), and *pseudofolliculitis barbae* have changes in keratinization and hyperkeratosis in their pathogenesis.

These are common indications for chemoexfoliation. But peel products are not interchangeable. Each chemical type has what it does better than the others or only does — we discuss this in the separate sections on the individual categories of peels.

Peels are used not only to remove aesthetic flaws in large areas of the face, neck, décolletage, and hands but also for therapeutic purposes. People suffering from ichthyosis have been shown to benefit from regular chemoexfoliation with polyhydroxy acids. By spot cauterization with keratolytic formulations, local defects (e.g., keratomas and warts) are destroyed. Today, chemical peels are successfully integrated into aesthetic programs along with injections and physical treatments, allowing us to achieve excellent results with minimal risk.

Interest in peels has increased dramatically since the concept of photoaging was formulated. According to this concept, most age-related skin changes (e.g., wrinkles, keratoses, age spots, telangiectasias) are indeed the result of damage to the skin by UV radiation and can be eliminated. Chemical peeling has proven to be not only effective but also a convenient way to combat the signs of photoaging because it does not require expensive equipment and can be easily accomplished in a cosmetic salon.

1.1.2. General contraindications

Inflammation is an absolute contraindication for any chemical peeling. Inflammation can be caused by various factors (e.g., disease, infection, trauma). If present, chemical peeling must not be performed in the affected area.

Peeling is contraindicated for **reactive (sensitive) skin** in cases of **individual intolerance** to the substances of the formulation. In addition, each chemical peel type has a specific list of contraindications which are discussed in specific chapters.

1.2. Biological basis

1.2.1. Chemical peeling is based on the skin's ability to renew itself

Usually, the rate of division of basal keratinocytes is equal to the corneocyte exfoliation (desquamation) rate. A complete cell turnover takes approximately 28 days to complete (so-called **physiological regeneration**). However, after a skin injury, the number of cell mitoses in the basal layer increases, the newly formed keratinocytes start moving faster up and sideways, and their maturation is also accelerated. This process occurs because the skin must close the "gap in the barrier" as soon as possible (so-called **physiological reparation**).

Epidermal regeneration and repair have much in common. They are realized due to the genetically determined changes (differentiation) of a keratinocyte on its life path, which begins in the basal layer and ends in the *stratum corneum*.

Any effect on the skin aiming at structural reorganization must rely on the skin's capacity for self-renewal. The deeper the lesion, the greater the load on the skin's repair systems and the greater the chance that something in the repair process can go wrong. Although a more aggressive peel may achieve greater skin renewal, you should assess the risks and try to match the depth of damage to the skin repairing capabilities before choosing it. For example, the older a person is, the poorer their repair systems are, so the more cautious we should be about treatment that damages the skin. The same applies to people suffering from a somatic disease or unstable psycho-emotional state: their resistance to aggressive external factors is reduced, and their recovery resources are depleted.

1.2.2. Epidermis, the primary target for chemical peels

The first question the professional must answer before starting the chemical peeling is: What exactly and to what extent should be destroyed?

The main impact of chemical peeling is on the epidermis. This is understandable because it is where the peel preparation is applied, and the chemical substances first react with the epidermal structures. The echoes of these reactions reach the dermal layer, which reacts to them (or does not react). Still, these are only echoes of the processes unfolding in the epidermis where the primary targets for peeling agents are located.

The peels' active components penetrate to different depths and interact with the skin structures differently. All peeling agents used today, except retinol, "act" through damage, directly destroying their target or disrupting its functioning. Accordingly, the more profound the targets are, the more serious the trauma caused to the skin during the procedure.

The following **factors** determine the degree of damage to the skin during chemical peeling:
- Chemical nature of the peeling agent
- Concentration of the peeling agent
- pH value of the applied preparation (for acid peels)
- Carrier, i.e., substances of the peel formulation enhancing the penetration of the peeling agent through the *stratum corneum*
- Exposure duration
- Skin condition at the site of peel application

Chemical peeling is classified according to **the impact depth**:
1. **Exfoliation** (the most superficial peeling) — accelerates the desquamation of the most superficial corneocytes, which are ready to leave the skin but remain on its surface (e.g., because of the "glue" composed of sebum, dust, and cosmetics). Often, exfoliation is the first (preparatory) step of cosmetic treatment.
2. **Superficial peeling** (at the *stratum corneum* level) — disintegrates corneodesmosomes, affecting the activity of enzymes in forming the lipid barrier and proteolytic destruction of corneodesmosomes.
3. **Superficial/medium-depth peeling** — has an effect up to the granular layer of the epidermis.
4. **Medium-depth peeling** — acts up to the basal layer of the epidermis.
5. **Deep peeling** — results in the removal of the epidermis, part of the growth zone, and the upper layers of the dermis that protrude into the epidermis (rete pegs).

The safest action is within the *stratum corneum*: most superficial corneocytes and dirt adhering to them are scrubbed off, and the skin's surface is smoothed without affecting the underlying living cells. Often, such polishing is enough to noticeably refresh the skin and give it a healthy and beautiful shine. Suppose the action is at the *stratum corneum* level (exfoliation and superficial peeling) and/or proceeds without damaging living cells (retinol peeling). In that case, the cosmetic treatment is one of the routine skincare stages and/or serves to prepare the skin for a further stronger peel and can be performed both in the aesthetic salon and at home.

If the chemical peeling damages living cells, it is classified as a medical treatment and must be performed in a medical office. Pain, swelling, extended recovery time, unwanted side effects such as pigmentation disorders, and outcome unpredictability must be expected — this is the price of the deep chemical peeling, which is inevitably accompanied by severe damage to the epidermal barrier. Fortunately, today we have an excellent alternative for dealing with deep skin structures in the form of cosmetic injections and physical treatments that minimally traumatize or do not traumatize the epidermis (Starkman S.J., Mangat D.S., 2020).

1.2.3. Chemical peeling "inside-out" and "outside-in": what's the difference?

Often (but not always) after peeling the skin begins to scale. The clinical picture (e.g., beginning and duration of the active phase, size and shape of the scales, scaling intensity) depends on the following:

- Depth and degree of the skin damage
- Chemical nature of the peeling agent
- Skin condition
- General health status

We have already mentioned that physiological skin exfoliation due to keratinocyte turnover occurs continuously, but if the skin is healthy, we do not notice the exfoliation. Visible scaling is a universal skin response to damage. Damaged skin tries to eliminate the destroyed elements as soon as possible. It sheds them off, making room for new, functionally active ones. The effect of peeling agents such as phenol, trichloroacetic acid, salicylic acid, α-hydroxy acids, and proteolytic enzymes is through damage. **Peeling performed**

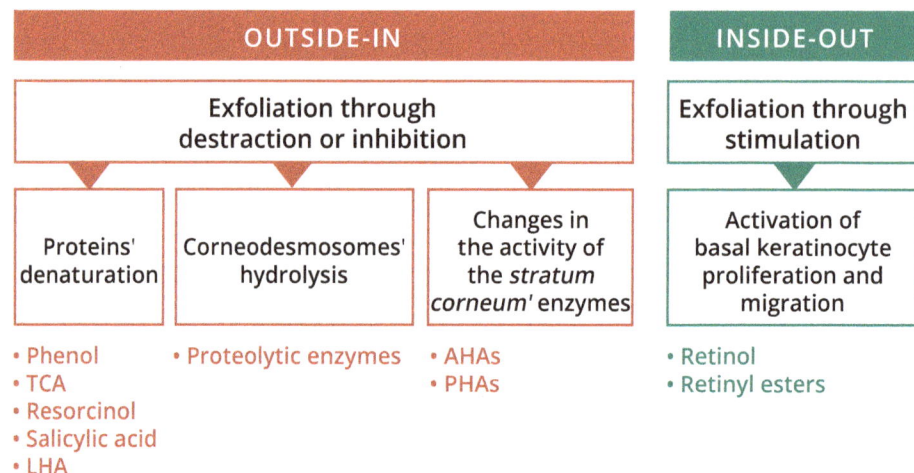

Figure I-2. Chemical peeling "outside-in" and "inside-out": the principle of action and peeling agents

through destabilizing effects on the *stratum corneum* is called "outside-in."

However, skin desquamation can be caused not only by damaging the skin barrier structures. Recall that the basal keratinocyte division rate is usually related to the corneocyte desquamation rate. If the rate of division is increased by stimulating mitosis, the newly formed cells move to the surface faster, as if displacing the overlying cell layers. Eventually, there is a mass reset of corneocytes on top, which become visible to the naked eye. This is how retinol, also used as a peeling agent, works. **Retinol triggers exfoliation by stimulating the division of basal keratinocytes. Because the *stratum corneum* does not react to retinol, retinol peeling is called "inside-out."** According to this principle, all currently known peeling agents are divided into destroyers and stimulators.

Peeling agents differ in their chemical nature and mechanisms of action. There are four types of chemical peels (**Fig. I-2**):
1. Keratolytic peels
2. Acid peels
3. Enzymatic peels
4. Retinol peels

We consider the peculiarities of each group of peels in the next part.

Part II
Types of chemical peels

Chapter 1
Keratolytic peels

The first peeling agents for medical purposes were keratolytic substances. Phenol, trichloroacetic acid, salicylic acid, and resorcinol have been used to treat scars and pigment spots since the 1880s. The term "keratolytic" was coined to describe the action of these compounds, which means "dissolver of horny scales" (from the Greek κέρατο — horn).

This name was given because when keratolytic substances were applied to the skin, a whitish plaque appeared on the surface, which was then easily washed off. Most plaque is built up of modified corneocytes filled with keratin. But keratin is not the only target for keratolytic agents, so in addition to their exfoliating effect, they are also characterized by other effects.

1.1. Features of keratolytic peels

1.1.1. Mechanism of action

Keratolytic agents react with proteins to **break the disulfide bonds** between the sulfur atoms of the amino acid cysteine (**Fig. II-1-1**). A covalent bond formed between two cysteines on one amino acid chain is called intramolecular while that formed on different chains is denoted as intermolecular.

With the help of disulfide bonds, a protein (or a protein complex, if it is composed of several chains) maintains a particular 3D configuration. Such a protein is called **native**, and only in native form it can perform the functions assigned to it, whether structural, enzymatic, or otherwise. As a result of breaking the stabilizing bonds, the protein unfolds and turns into an amino acid chain — a **denatured** protein that is no longer functional.

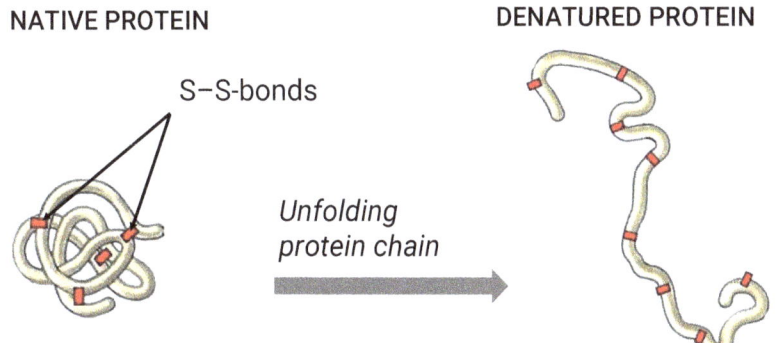

Figure II-1-1. Mechanism of keratolytic action: breaking of stabilizing disulfide bonds (–S–S–) in a protein molecule or protein complex

1.1.2. Skin targets for keratolytic agents

Keratolytics interact with ALL proteins stabilized by disulfide bonds, i.e., their action is not selective and is not limited to keratin. In addition to keratin, other proteins in the *stratum corneum* and epidermis can also be denatured when encountering a keratolytic agent, affecting the clinical result.

Skin surface
All keratolytics are antiseptics. They chemically modify **the proteins of the shells of microorganisms** (e.g., bacteria, fungi, and even viruses) in the area of application. If the wall damage is extensive, the microorganism dies.

The *stratum corneum* contains the following keratolytic targets (**Fig. II-1-2**):
- **Corneocyte proteins** — keratin (inside the corneocytes) and the cornified envelope proteins*
- **Corneodesmosomes** — protein bridges that bind corneocytes together and maintain the integrity of the *stratum corneum*

---

* The corneocytes are surrounded by a proteinaceous structure called the cornified envelope. This structure consists of a layer of highly cross-linked insoluble proteins covalently bound to a layer of lipids.

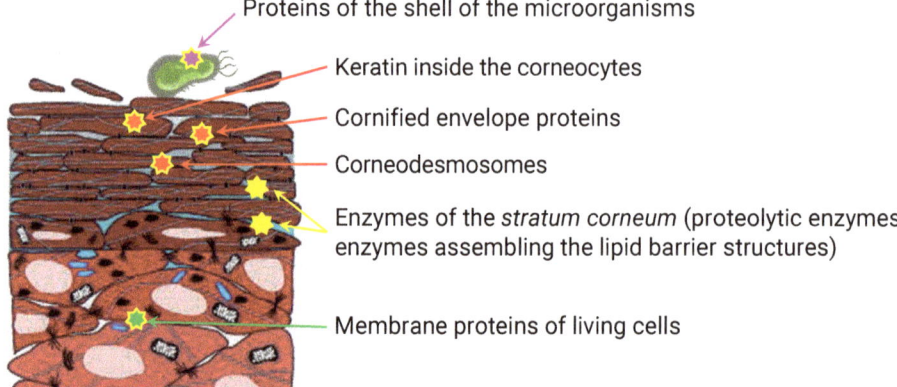

Figure II-1-2. Targets for keratolytic agents

- **Enzymes** — proteolytic enzymes (they "cut" the corneodesmosomes and are responsible for desquamation) and enzymes assembling the lipid barrier between the corneocytes

Living layers

What happens if the substance passes through the *stratum corneum* and ends up in the living cells' territory? The same process occurs — the keratolytic agent reacts chemically with the proteins, damaging their structure. The greatest danger to living cells is damage to **the cell membrane proteins that form the pores** — if they are denatured, the membrane ceases to filter the flow of substances entering and leaving the cell, and the cell quickly dies. All living cells — not only keratinocytes but also melanocytes, immunocytes, and skin receptors — are defenseless against keratolytic agents.

A person feels **pain** when a keratolytic agent enters the epidermis, which is attributed to the chemical damage to the membrane proteins of the skin receptors. To get rid of the damaging substance, living cells release various mediators, including vasodilators, to accelerate blood flow to the area and ensure the dissolution and excretion of the keratolytic agent. Therefore, erythema and edema indicate that the keratolytic agent has passed through the barrier and has reached the living cells.

Keratolytics are not selective — all cells in their path are attacked. This explains the inherent cytotoxicity of all keratolytic substances. Therefore, they should not be allowed to penetrate the *stratum corneum* without a strong reason.

1.1.3. Features of keratolytic peeling

Keratolytic peels have their peculiarities, both clinical and practical. All keratolytics are characterized by the appearance of the so-called **frost** on the skin during the procedure — a whitish plaque composed of denatured skin proteins.

Frost is an indication that the keratolytic agent has begun to work. In addition, it indicates the degree of skin damage (**Fig. II-1-3**). Thus, for TCA peeling, frost is used to control the reaction depth and determine when to stop the procedure. For phenol, dense frost appears quickly after the application.

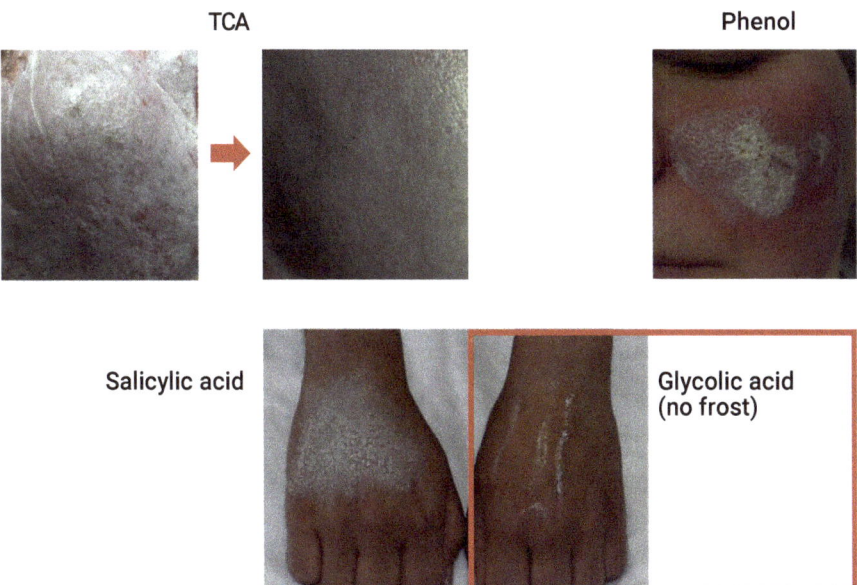

Figure II-1-3. Keratolytic peeling feature: whitish plaque on the skin (frost)

It is surrounded by erythema which is a sign of severe skin irritation. There is no redness during conventional superficial salicylic peeling, only a light plaque (unlike the frost with TCA and phenol, salicylic frost is sometimes called pseudo-frost, but it has the same origin and is composed of denatured proteins). There may be mild redness with superficial/medium-depth frost. In comparison, when treating with other peeling agents (AHAs, enzymes, retinol), there is no frost because there is no protein denaturation. These agents have different mechanisms of action, as we will explain in the corresponding sections.

The degree and speed of skin damage depend on:
1. Concentration of the keratolytic in the preparation — the higher it is, the more extensive the damage
2. Exposure duration — the longer it is, the more extensive the damage
3. Condition of the *stratum corneum* — the thinner it is, the greater the chances for substances to pass through it and get to the living layers

Depending on these parameters, the damage can be superficial (at the level of the *stratum corneum*) or deeper, affecting the living layers of the epidermis. **Unlike acid peels, keratolytic peels do not need to be neutralized.** The keratolytic mechanism is based on a chemical reaction with proteins independent of the pH value. To stop the keratolytic action and remove it from the skin, it is necessary to wash the skin thoroughly with water or a special solution that removes poorly water-soluble substances, which include keratolytics.

Keratolytic substances vary in ability to penetrate the *stratum corneum* and toxicity levels. Phenol and TCA are the most hazardous, and despite being prohibited in the cosmetics industry, they can still be found on the gray market.

We hope that the information presented in our book will serve as a warning to those who continue to use phenol and TCA in their practice and make them think about whether it is worth risking the health of their patients for no good reason (Wambier C.G. et al., 2019).

1.2. Trichloroacetic acid

Trichloroacetic acid (CCl$_3$COOH) is a fully halogenated (by methyl group) analog of acetic acid. It is soluble in water, acetone, benzene, methylene chloride, and carbon disulfide. It is strongly toxic, can be absorbed through the skin, and has a cauterizing effect. It has a pleasant odor, which may be misleading.

The first knowledge about the effect of trichloroacetic acid (TCA) on the skin was obtained empirically. At first, dermatologists used TCA to treat skin diseases (for local cauterization), then aestheticians recognized its potential to eliminate aesthetic flaws.

1.2.1. Mechanism of action

TCA denatures skin proteins by breaking disulfide bonds. Painful sensations accompany the TCA peeling. The degree of damage is determined by frost, a grayish-white plaque composed of coagulated proteins that appears after some time on the area of TCA application (**Fig. II-1-4**).

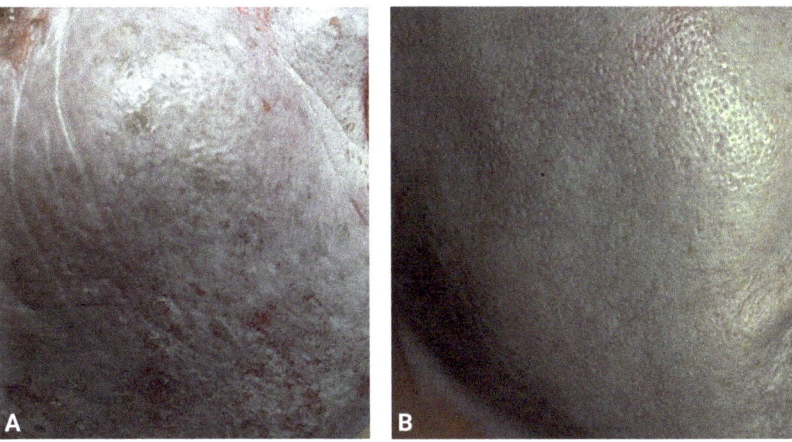

Figure II-1-4. Frost during TCA peeling: (A) first white-pink, then white, and then (B) dense grayish–white

The main problem with TCA peels, as with phenol peels, is controlling the depth and ensuring even penetration of the peeling agent. In this regard, the result of the procedure depends not only on the peeling agent itself but also on the specialist's skill. Although frost correlates with the degree of skin damage, it is not always possible to grasp its appearance and intensity (**Table II-1-1**).

Table II-1-1. Frost and degree of skin damage for TCA peeling

FROST	CLINICAL SIGNS	DEGREE OF DAMAGE
Level 0 No frost	Skin may look like it is lightly salted and shiny, but there is no solid plaque, no erythema	• Superficial peeling, affecting the *stratum corneum* • Barrier function is restored in 1–2 days
Level 1 Uneven light frost	Skin is shiny; erythema is clearly visible; some areas of skin have white spots of frost	• Superficial/medium-depth peeling, affecting the *stratum granulosum* • Healing takes 2–4 days
Level 2 White frost with pink streaks	Skin is covered with uniform white plaque, but there is a bright pink background	• Medium-depth peeling, affecting the *stratum spinosum* • Healing takes about 5 days
Level 3 Dense gray–white frost	Skin is covered with a dense layer of gray–white plaque without a pink background	• Medium-depth/deep peeling; skin damage is possible up to the basal membrane • Healing takes about 7 days

The first person who managed to create a reliable method for determining the depth of TCA penetration was the American dermatologist Zein Obagi. He compared the histological picture of skin damage with clinical signs and developed the criteria for assessing the TCA penetration depth (Johnson J.B. et al., 1996; Obagi Z.E. et al., 1999). As a result of these studies, the famous Blue Peel, in which TCA is mixed with a unique blue base, appeared on the market. The peel product must be applied layer by layer (the number of layers depends on the desired degree of damage — from superficial to medium-depth), staining the skin blue. On the one hand, the blue base slows down the TCA passage, preventing it from quickly "falling" under the *stratum corneum*. It changes the skin color depending on the TCA penetration depth. Frost appears faster and more clearly on the blue background, making the skin areas where TCA has penetrated deeper (looking like lighter spots) more readily apparent.

Besides the Blue Peel, there are other TCA peel systems on the market with a color indicator of the penetration depth, e.g., Peelosophy (Christina, Israel). However, in this case, the indicator is yellow. Before application on the skin, the TCA solution is mixed with a special preparation (the so-called evaluator), which slows down the penetration of TCA through the *stratum corneum* and turns the treated skin areas yellow. Whitish spots of frost gradually appear on the yellow skin, signaling that coagulation of proteins in the epidermal living layers has occurred.

1.2.2. Safety aspects

Compared to phenol peeling, TCA peeling is less aggressive and less risky, as well as less painful, but is more painful than acid peeling. Clinical observations indicate that TCA can be used for superficial and medium-depth peeling, while the risk of complications is too high for deep peeling (if TCA concertation exceeds 40%). The depth of damage, healing time, and complete skin color recovery depend on the TCA concentration and thickness of the *stratum corneum* and epidermis.

Complications after TCA peeling are the same as those after phenol peeling, although they occur to a much lesser extent. Nonetheless, peeling is a severe challenge to the skin and the body, so the patient's physical and psychological readiness for this treatment is important.

There are several **absolute** and **relative contraindications** that need to be considered before proceeding with TCA peeling:
- Warts on the face
- Abnormal skin reaction to a previous chemical peeling or dermabrasion
- Herpes
- Photosensitivity

- Skin phototype V–VI
- Radiation therapy in connection with cancer
- Keloid or hypertrophic scars
- Pregnancy, lactation
- Roaccutane/Accutane (isotretinoin) administration six months before and six months after chemical peeling (the literature describes cases of scar formation in those who started taking isotretinoin after the peeling)
- Intensive exposure to sunlight at least two days before the peeling
- Surgery or cryosurgery in the treatment area (at least six weeks before the peeling)

1.2.3. Practical aspects

The TCA peels are divided into three groups:
1. 20% TCA — for superficial peeling
2. 20–40% TCA — for medium-depth peeling
3. Over 40% TCA — for the destruction of local defects

Adhering to the following rules significantly increases the chance of success:
- Stop using sponges and scrubs 3–4 weeks before the procedure
- Do not wax the area you plan to treat 4 weeks before the procedure
- Do not shave the treatment area the day before the procedure
- Two weeks before peel treatment, apply AHA-containing cream (3–8%) at night to soften the skin and weaken the corneocyte cohesion

Brody H.J. and Hailey C.W. (1986) suggested that, to improve the uniformity of TCA penetration, the skin should be cooled with artificial ice for 5–10 seconds, after which a 35% TCA solution should be applied. According to these authors, preliminary "freezing" increases skin permeability and allows for more uniform acid penetration.

Monheit proposed another technique in the 1980s. First, the skin is treated with a Jessner solution (14% lactic acid, 14% salicylic acid, 14% resorcinol) to loosen the bonds between corneocytes, and then a 35% TCA peel solution is applied. As a result, TCA penetration becomes more uniform (Monheit G.D., 1989). Coleman W.P. and Futrell J.M. (1994) demonstrated that a similar result could be achieved by pre-treating the skin with 70% glycolic acid followed by 35% TCA. Most modern TCA peels have a gel base, which is advantageous for two reasons: it provides a more even distribution of the product on the skin and allows for a slower and more gradual diffusion of TCA molecules into the skin.

If TCA is used to cauterize local skin imperfections such as warts or post-acne scars, the procedure is much easier than treating large areas. One to three drops of 40–100% TCA is applied to cleansed skin, avoiding neighboring areas. After frost appears (in about 20–30 minutes), the area should be treated with a special ointment or petroleum jelly. In about a week, the skin on the treated area sloughs (Lee J.B. et al., 2002). If necessary, the procedure can be repeated after 1–3 months (**Fig. II-1-5**). This method is known as the chemical reconstruction of skin scars (CROSS).

Even after the careful implementation of the physician's recommendations before and after the peel treatment and a skillfully executed procedure, undesirable skin reactions can still occur. For example, during the first week after the peel procedure, the skin may

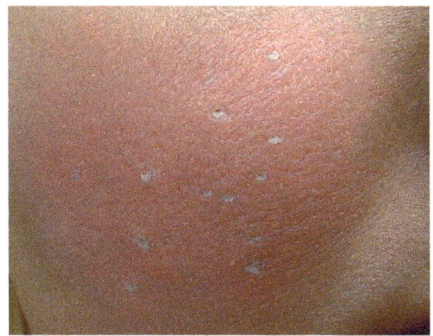
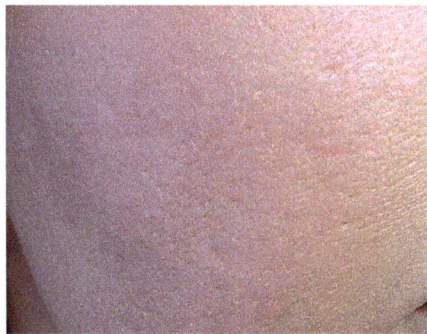

65–100% TCA, spot cauterization — After 12 treatments

Figure II-1-5. Spot cauterization of post-acne scars with a highly concentrated TCA preparation (CROSS)

remain red and swollen, you may feel a burning sensation, and there may be a serous exudate. Sometimes after chemical peeling, the skin remains red for a long time and, in rare cases, depigmentation may occur. The most common side effect is the appearance of brown spots (the so-called bronzing effect). This phenomenon is reversible, although the spots remain for a long time. As the spots occur if the skin has been exposed to sunlight after TCA peeling, it is necessary to use sunscreens with the sun protection factor (SPF) of at least 25. If the patient has herpes, chemical peeling can provoke its exacerbation. Hence, it is recommended to take lysine-containing supplements two weeks before the treatment as prevention.

In contrast to phenol peeling, TCA peeling can be performed more than once. The interval between treatments depends on the depth of the peel: it should be several months for superficial peels, and up to one year for medium-depth peels. **Currently, TCA is prohibited for use in skincare practice in most countries.**

1.2.4. Modified TCA for chemical skin remodeling

Despite the ban on TCA in skincare products, it is too early to cross the substance out of the cosmetic arsenal: TCA is back but in a modified form. A few years ago, a product containing TCA in a complex with urea peroxide was launched. Being a part of the complex, TCA is not active and does not destroy proteins. The complex is relatively stable, but once decomposed it, releases TCA, urea, and peroxide, which quickly decomposes to water and oxygen.

Interestingly, the complex quickly passes through the *stratum corneum* and epidermis and reaches the dermis. Most of the complexes disintegrate in the dermal layer via the following process. TCA nonselectively denatures protein structures, including "old" fibers, making them available for destruction by metalloproteinases and subsequent replacement by new fibers, while oxygen intensifies cellular respiration and synthetic activity of fibroblasts. A small part of free TCA released in the epidermis is enough to stimulate the division and migration of basal keratinocytes. However, this effect is incomparable with the extensive damage to the barrier structures and epidermis observed during medium-depth TCA peeling (Buslaeva E.R., 2016).

Immediately after the treatment, there is an increase in skin turgor, straightening of superficial wrinkles, and a slight blush that gives a fresh look. This is due to the reaction of the skin vessels: they expand, providing blood flow to the treatment site. This effect can be observed for several days. A moisturizer may easily correct slight flaking a few days after the procedure. There are two versions of modified TCA treatment: one using a TCA/urea peroxide complex and the other using trichloroacetate ammonium (TCAA) with hydrogen peroxide. The TCA/peroxide complex is more stable. Compared to the TCA/urea peroxide ammonium complex, it does not hydrolyze as quickly, which is safer due to the slower release of TCA and prolongs the action of the substance in the skin (Shai A.M., 2019).

In preparations for chemical remodeling, the concentration of modified TCA can be as high as 35%, which is equivalent to the TCA concentration for medium-depth peel. TCA modification minimizes the risks of side effects. It offers a fundamentally new procedure, which in its indications (laxity, atrophic scars, striae, post-acne scars) and clinical effects (thickening and lifting) is closer to remodeling techniques than peels. This peculiarity is reflected in its name: Chemical Remodeling Technology (Korneeva R.V., Voytenko I.V., 2019).

After chemical remodeling, there is no need for a recovery period. The procedures can be performed year-round. They can be recommended as an express procedure "for going out." In addition, they are suitable for preparing the skin for aggressive aesthetic procedures, prolonging and enhancing the effect of injections and physical treatments.

1.3. Phenol

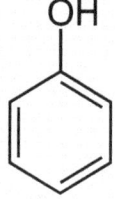

Phenols (C_6H_5OH, oxybenzene, commonly referred to as carbolic acid) are colorless needle-like crystals that turn pink in the air due to oxidation, resulting in the coloring of products containing this compound. They have a specific odor of gouache. Soluble in water (6 g per 100 g of water), alkaline solutions, alcohol, benzene, and acetone.

During World War I, La Gasse, a French physician, noticed that treating wounds with carbolic acid made the skin lighter, smoother, and more uniform. After the war, his daughter Antoinette brought the technique of phenol peeling to the U.S., where she began a private cosmetic practice. Soon phenol peeling became very popular among aestheticians in Florida and California. At that time, aestheticians were in no hurry to reveal the formulations of their preparations, and carefully guarded their "secret formulas" from other practitioners.

In 1961, Litton, an American physician, demonstrated to the medical community the results of phenol peeling in 50 patients. Litton bought the peel formula containing 50% phenol, glycerin, and croton oil (Asian *Croton tiglium* oil with irritating properties) from an aesthetician who successfully used it in practice. In 1962, Litton published his observations but kept the formula private. The same happened with the dermatologist Brown, who patented the formula containing croton oil and phenol (also obtained by him from aestheticians) in 1959 but did not specify the full formulation.

Eventually, all the glory went to Baker and Gordon from Miami, FL, who, having obtained the recipe of phenol peel, made it public in 1961. The Baker–Gordon formula included 3 ml of 88% phenol, 2 ml of distilled water, eight drops of liquid Septisol soap, and three drops of croton oil. Baker believed that diluted phenol penetrates deeper into the skin than undiluted phenol (most likely because undiluted phenol denatures the *stratum corneum* proteins too quickly with the formation of large aggregates, which slows further phenol penetration into the skin).

The Baker–Gordon formula became the standard for phenol peels. Yet, despite using it for many years, none of the dermatologists referred in their works to the aestheticians from whom they obtained the formula. The truth was revealed later when the coryphaei of dermatology began to share their memories.

Eventually, the practice of phenol peeling primarily passed from the hands of aestheticians to physicians. Numerous lawsuits against aestheticians practicing phenol peeling forced most of them to stop using the technique.

1.3.1. Mechanism of action

Phenol is a very poisonous substance that is easily and quickly absorbed by the skin. In the *stratum corneum*, phenol breaks disulfide bonds of protein components (keratin and corneodesmosomes), leading to their denaturation. The complex of denatured proteins with phenol penetrates through the *stratum corneum* slower because it is big and less soluble in the lipids that fill the intercellular spaces of the *stratum corneum*.

Phenol is like fire indiscriminately burning out everything in its path. It is not easy to control the destructive power of phenol, so the risk of complications is high. Penetrating under the *stratum corneum*, phenol reacts with all intercellular and cellular protein structures on its way (e.g., proteins of the intercellular matrix, basal membrane, and cell surface receptors). When phenol reacts with receptors of nerve endings in the skin, a person feels pain.

In the skin exposed to phenol, changes are observed at the level of reticular derma: collagen and elastin pattern in the treated areas changes — it becomes more flattened, with fibrous elements parallel to the skin surface. At the same time, the dermis becomes thicker and denser. The new state of the derma is relatively stable and lasts for a long time, and outwardly it is reflected in a much smoother skin microrelief.

The first studies on the effectiveness of phenol peeling were clinical observations, but were soon followed by analyses of morphological changes in the skin. In 1985, Kligman, Baker, and Gordon showed that:

1. Phenol in the Baker–Gordon formula penetrates the skin much better than undiluted phenol.
2. Up to 3 mm thick layers of "fresh" elastin are found in the skin that has undergone phenol peeling.

Subsequent experiments led to some conclusions that are essential for practical applications. For example, it was shown that the degree of visible desquamation without occlusion coating would be relatively weak. Occlusion improves phenol penetration. Adding a small amount of croton oil significantly increases the visible scaling and prolongs the healing period.

According to the classification by Hetter, the degree of phenol peeling is determined by the time needed for subsequent recovery:
- Light — 5 days
- Moderate — 7 days
- Moderate/intense — 10–14 days

Hetter modified the Baker–Gordon formula, adapting it for different needs (**Table II-1-2**). He published the results of his research in 2000, triggering a new wave of interest in phenol peeling (Hetter G.P., 2000a,b,c,d). The main difference between Hetter's formulas and the Baker–Gordon formula is the amount of croton oil. Hetter showed a positive link between croton oil content and the degree of skin scaling, and suggested several formulations. According to Hetter, the safety level of these formulations is higher. Moreover, the "lightest" formula can be used even in highly delicate areas such as around the eyes (Larson D.L. et al., 2009).

Before, during, and after the phenol treatment, a patient must drink plenty of water — up to two liters per day. Sedation (alprazolam, zolpidem, and ibuprofen/oxycodone) eight hours before the treatment is mandatory.

1.3.2. Safety aspects

Despite the advent of safer modified phenol formulations, high phenol toxicity remains a severe problem, especially for people with heart, liver, and kidney disorder (Downs J.W., Wills B.K., 2020).

Table II-1-2. Modified Baker–Gordon formulas (Hetter's formulas)

BAKER–GORDON FORMULA	HETTER'S FORMULAS			
Skin scaling				
Very intensive	Light/moderate (for general use)	Very light (for the eye and neck area)	Moderate/intensive	Intensive
Phenol/Croton oil (%/% vol)				
50/2.1	33/0.35	27.5/0.105	33/0.7	33/1.1
Composition				
• Phenol 88% (3 ml) • Water (2 ml) • Septisol (8 drops) • Croton oil (3 drops)	• Phenol 88% (4 ml) • Water (6 ml) • Liquid soap (16 drops) • Croton oil (one drop)	Take 3 ml of the mild to moderate peel formula and add: • Phenol 88% (2 ml) • Water (5 ml)	• Phenol 88% (4 ml) • Water (6 ml) • Liquid soap (16 drops) • Croton oil (2 drops)	• Phenol 88% (4 ml) • Water (6 ml) • Liquid soap (16 drops) • Croton oil (3 drops)

The toxic effect of phenol, manifested by arrhythmia, occurs when a specific concentration of phenol in the blood is reached. The lethal phenol concentration is 23 mg/100 ml of blood.

Phenol is a compound familiar to the human organism. When microflora enzymes break down tyrosine in the gut, phenol and cresol are formed, so the organism knows how to neutralize phenol and get rid of it. After absorption into the blood from the intestine, phenol enters the liver, where enzyme systems modify it into harmless and water-soluble compounds, which are then eliminated from the body by the kidneys. Thanks to its well-established utilization, phenol does not accumulate in the body, so there should be no delayed toxicity.

Phenol concentration in the blood during the treatment depends on its absorption rate through the skin and the degradation rate in the body. Since phenol is absorbed through the skin and does not enter the liver immediately, its concentration in the blood during the procedure will be determined by the following factors:

- Total phenol amount applied to the skin (it should also be considered that the lower the concentration of phenol, the easier it penetrates the skin)
- Frequency of the phenol formulation application
- Rate of phenol transdermal absorption and transformation in the body
- The larger the surface area to be treated, the faster the phenol enters the bloodstream (for example, a quick treatment of the entire body with a 2% phenol solution can be fatal because too much phenol would immediately enter the bloodstream)

If the phenol solution is applied slowly, the liver would have time to neutralize the phenol, and the risk of poisoning would be reduced.

The absolute **contraindications** to phenol peeling are:

- Liver, kidney, and cardiovascular disorders
- Pregnancy, lactation
- Cancer of any etiology
- Chronic skin diseases (e.g., psoriasis, atopic dermatitis, ichthyosis)
- Autoimmune diseases
- Inflammatory dermatoses
- Eczema
- Skin phototype IV–VI

Elderly patients fall into a group with an increased risk. First, the resource of health and functional activity of internal organs decreases with age: the activity of neutralizing enzyme systems in the liver and the rate of phenol metabolite excretion by the kidneys decrease. Second, patients of this age may regularly take a few medications (e.g., aspirin), which are also neutralized by liver enzymes. If so, toxic poisoning may occur due to the accumulation of untreated carbolic acid in the body. Another risk factor is that the course of the phenol peeling is not easy to predict, given that phenol absorption through the skin varies from person to person.

The damage caused by phenol peeling is comparable to 3rd-degree burns. In the case of extensive damage, a burn disease develops. The observed **adverse events** and **complications** can be divided into two categories (Brody H.J., 2018):
1. Life-threatening: heart attacks, arrhythmias, kidney failure
2. Non-life-threatening: atypical spots, increased allergic reactions, herpes exacerbation, scarring (in case of trauma or infection in the post-operative period), whitehead acne, and infection

One of the permanent consequences of phenol peeling is the disruption in the activity of pigment-producing cells, the melanocytes. Even if the procedure is performed without destroying the melanocytes, their ability to produce pigment is permanently reduced, and the patient's face takes on a characteristic porcelain hue. The area treated with phenol sometimes contrasts sharply with the rest of the skin: a clear border (demarcation line) appears between treated and untreated areas, and this undesirable effect is especially noticeable in patients with dark skin. For example, after local peel around the mouth, there may be a "clown face," and when the entire face is peeled, there may be a "white mask."

Another common complication of phenol peeling is skin darkening. The risk of hyperpigmentation is especially high in dark skin, so phenol peeling is contraindicated in people with dark or black skin. Patients with adrenal insufficiency also have a predisposition to hyperpigmentation. After a deep phenol peeling, the skin loses the ability to produce pigment properly. This is an irreversible process.

After phenol peeling, patients must protect their skin from the sun for life and need to use sunscreens with UV filters at all times of the year. Disregarding these recommendations is likely to result in not only the appearance of pigment spots but also serious pathologies (including skin cancer). Quite unpleasant and frequent complications of phenol peeling are the formation of keloid and hypertrophic scars, as well as skin atrophy.

1.3.3. Practical aspects

Phenol peeling requires adherence to specific rules.
1. During the treatment, the patient must be connected to a heart monitor. This allows the physician to notice signs of cardiac abnormality in time and stop the procedure. Patients with liver pathology and cardiovascular and kidney disorders should never be given phenol peeling.
2. To reduce the concentration of phenol in the blood and accelerate its elimination from the body, the patient is given plenty of fluids before the procedure, and intravenous infusions of glucose solution are often carried out during the procedure.
3. Phenol peeling is an excruciating procedure, so anesthesia is required.

The phenol peel formulation must be applied slowly and gradually so that the liver has time to break down the phenol in the blood. Usually, the face is divided into areas not exceeding 25% of its surface, and 15-minute breaks are taken between treatments.

After deep phenol peeling, the skin recovers within three weeks. The recovery is usually accompanied by significant swelling. Crust detachment is usually observed in the third week, and pronounced hyperemia persists for up to one month. Complete recovery of the skin color lasts about six months.

Long rehabilitation and many contraindications make phenol peeling unattractive for patients. Nevertheless, there are still studies aimed at finding ways to prevent the toxic effects of phenol (especially the potentially lethal ones, such as cardiac arrhythmia) and facilitate more accurate control of the penetration depth (Hetter G.P., 2000a–d; Sun H.F. et al., 2018; Justo A.D.S. et al., 2020). The latter is needed because overly deep skin necrosis results in complications, such as scarring, pigmentation disorders (hypo- and hyper-), and persistent skin reddening.

Phenol peeling can be done once in a lifetime, as it may leave behind permanent structural changes in the skin that are not always desirable. Considering that, in cosmetic dermatology, there are now many other safer and more effective methods to reconstruct deep layers of the skin, using phenol peel is rarely advised. Finally, given the ban on its use in skincare, which is justified, **phenol peeling has become illegal**.

1.4. Salicylic acid and lipohydroxy acid (LHA)

Salicylic acid (2-hydroxybenzoic acid), $C_6H_4(OH)COON$ is a colorless crystalline substance, well soluble in ethanol, diethyl ether, and other polar organic solvents, and poorly soluble in water (1.8 g/l at 20 °C).

Salicylic acid was first isolated from the willow bark (*Salix L.*). It is also found in other plant sources, such as birch bark and gaultheria leaves. Salicylic acid is a phenol molecule with an additional carboxy group. It has hydroxy and carboxy groups, which is why salicylic acid is classified as a hydroxy acid (see Part II, chapter 2). This classification confuses aestheticians and ordinary cosmetics users, who put salicylic acid in line with glycolic acid, lactic acid, tartaric acid, and other alpha hydroxy acids (AHAs).

The chemical properties of salicylic acid have nothing in common with water-soluble AHAs, but **they are very close to those of phenol**. First, salicylic acid is poorly soluble in water. For this reason, unlike water-soluble AHAs, it is unaffected by the the pH value (reflecting the concentration of hydrogen ions in a water solution). Second, salicylic acid can react with disulfide bonds, while AHAs cannot, so their molecular mechanism of action is fundamentally different from the keratolytic one (see Part II, section 2.1).

Salicylic acid is often added to cosmetic products for oily skin. Due to its keratolytic action, it opens comedones, improving sebum evacuation from the sebaceous gland ducts.

The concentration of salicylic acid is quite variable:
- Leave-on cosmetic products: 0.5–1% (up to 2%)
- Rinse-off masks: 2–5%
- Peel formulations: 15–30%

Liposalicylic acid is 2-hydroxy-5-octanoylbenzoic acid (C8-β-lipohydroxy acid), a salicylic acid to which a fatty acid is attached. It is well soluble in fats and insoluble in water.

Lipohydroxy acid (LHA), a lipid derivative of salicylic acid, is known on the cosmetics market. The LHA molecule is larger and has a higher affinity to lipids, so it accumulates in the lipid layer of the *stratum corneum* and loosens it. Salicylic acid and LHA destroy corneodesmosomes in different ways. Salicylic acid is active across the entire thickness of the *stratum corneum*. LHA acts on the corneocytes located at a depth of the 3rd–4th layers of the *stratum corneum* — it is at this depth that the desquamation process begins. In contrast to the indiscriminate salicylic acid action, LHA selectively influences only the corneodesmosomes that have already started to undergo the process of enzymatic destruction. Finally, the nature of corneodesmosome destruction by LHA is different from that of salicylic acid: in the case of LHA, the protein bridges are more severely affected.

Additionally, LHA exhibits antimicrobial, fungicidal, anti-inflammatory, and comedolytic properties, which make this substance a highly influential component of soft peels, as well as preparations for oily skin, acne and post-acne treatment, and restoration of photodamaged skin. The LHA concentration in at-home peel products is 5–10%. The valid patent for LHA belongs to L'Oréal, so now it is found in the products of L'Oréal brands only.

Salicylic acid and LHA combine well with other peeling agents, acting synergistically with them. By gently exfoliating the *stratum*

IMMEDIATE	DELAYED
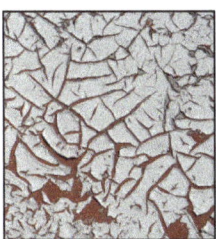 Frost Large flakes Permeability increase	 Fine flakes (possible)
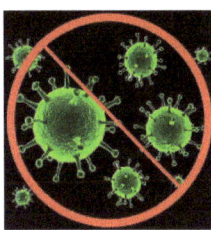 Antiseptic	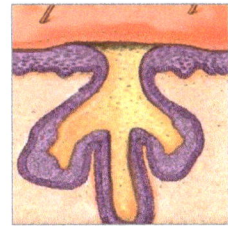 Reduction of skin oiliness

Figure II-1-6. Effects of salicylic peeling

corneum, they indirectly stimulate the division of basal keratinocytes. They are characterized by a high level of safety and are well tolerated even by sensitive skin. As a rule, the effects of salicylic acid and LHA are cumulative and require a series of treatments with products containing these compounds.

1.4.1. Mechanism of action and clinical effects

The clinical effects of salicylic peeling are divided into **rapid** (appearing during or immediately after the treatment) and **delayed** (**Fig. II-1-6**). In contact with the skin, salicylic acid quickly reacts with the *stratum corneum* proteins, especially corneodesmosomes and cornified envelopes proteins. It destroys them and provokes **immediate corneocyte desquamation**.

We see a white plaque (frost) and flakes during the procedure. The *stratum corneum* becomes loose, and its permeability increases. The **antiseptic effect** appears immediately after salicylic acid application. This is explained by the denaturation of proteins found in the shells of all microorganisms living on the skin surface in the treatment area.

However, **delayed desquamation** does not always occur. It is associated with damage to the *stratum corneum* enzymes responsible for its formation and renewal. If their work is disturbed, the structures that were formed deep in the *stratum corneum* at that moment are not properly built — the skin tends to "drop" them as soon as possible. Fine flaking a few days after salicylic peeling is indicative of such enzyme failure. However, this is not always the case for everyone and is usually related to the exposure time — the longer it is, the more likely it is that the salicylic acid will disrupt the enzymes.

All these are non-specific effects, typical of keratolytic agents in general. Apart from these, salicylic acid has a very important **specific effect**: being a small and oil-soluble molecule, it penetrates sebaceous glands filled with sebum quite easily, reaches sebocytes, and suppresses sebum lipid production. Moreover, it triggers the death of sebocytes by apoptosis, reducing the number of secretory cells in the sebaceous gland, which reduces the amount of sebum produced.

Recent studies have shed light on another known observation relating to the anti-inflammatory effect of salicylic formulations. It turns out that among the cytokines that sebocytes produce are pro-inflammatory mediators that trigger and maintain inflammation. Salicylic acid suppresses their production through the nuclear transcription factor NF-κB pathway, which controls the expression of the immune response, apoptosis, and cell cycle genes (Lu J. et al., 2019).

1.4.2. Indications and contraindications

Salicylic peeling is used to correct signs of chrono- and photoaging if the skin is not deficient in sebum. If the skin lacks sebum, preparations with salicylic acid are not recommended either for care or for peel. Accordingly, to treat age-related epidermal changes in dry, sebum-deficient skin, enzymatic or acidic peels should be used.

The anti-inflammatory effects of salicylic acid, supported by antiseptic, comedolytic, and anti-keratotic effects, render salicylic peeling particularly well suited for treating seborrhea and skin pathologies associated with increased sebum secretion (acne, seborrheic dermatitis, seborrheic keratosis) as well as psoriasis (**Fig. II-1-7**).

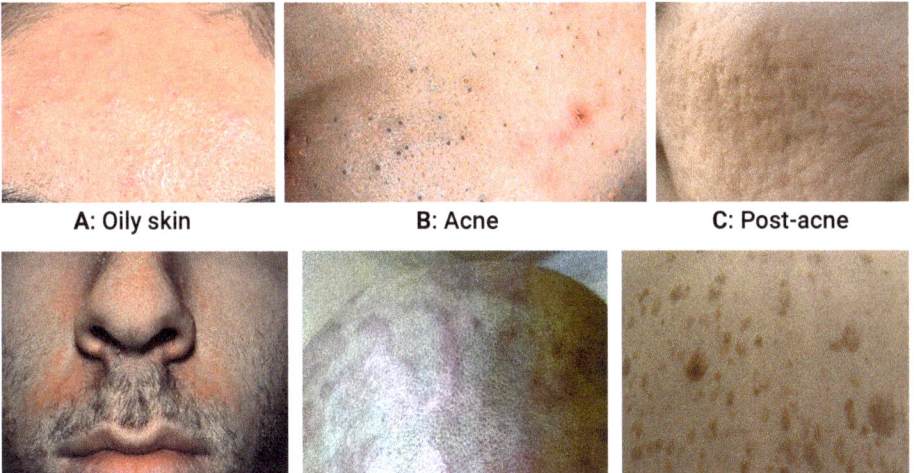

Figure II-1-7. Special indications for salicylic peeling
(Images by: A–C — Freepik.com, D, E — Wikipedia.com)

Indications for salicylic peeing:
- Epidermal age-related signs
- Photoaging
- Oily skin (seborrhea)
- Acne (non-inflammatory) and post-acne
- Seborrheic dermatitis
- Psoriasis
- Seborrheic keratosis (seborrheic keratoma)

Contraindications:
- Decreased sebaceous gland activity (lack of sebum)
- Atopic dermatitis
- Herpes in the active phase or with a recent exacerbation
- Hypersensitivity to salicylic acid
- Allergies to aspirin and salicylates
- Sunburns in the intended treatment area
- Pregnancy, lactation
- Less than two weeks after a laser or intense pulsed light (IPL) treatment

1.4.3. Practical aspects

No special conditions or special equipment are required for salicylic peeling. The product is applied to the cleansed skin with a fan brush and left for some time (10–15 minutes on average), then washed off with plenty of water after which a soothing and protective cream is applied.

Client should be advised not to wash their face for 24 hours after the superficial and 48 hours after the medium-depth peel. The rehabilitation period depends on the salicylic peeling intensity and the individual skin characteristics. On average, it takes about a week. During this time, it is necessary to use sunscreen and Panthenol can be applied to improve healing.

Salicylic peeling is a superficial peel that patients with any skin phototype tolerate well. A course usually includes 5–10 sessions at 7–14-day intervals. An aesthetician with a paramedical background can perform salicylic peeling. Cosmetic products containing salicylic acid can be used 1–2 times daily.

1.5. Resorcinol and Jessner peel

Resorcinol (resorcinol, 1,3-dihydroxybenzene, meta-dihydroxybenzene) is an organic compound with the formula $C_6H_4(OH)_2$, and has the physical appearance of colorless crystals with a peculiar odor. It differs in structure from hydroquinone only by the position of hydroxyl groups.

Resorcinol, another phenol derivative with keratolytic properties, is much less common in skincare practice than salicylic acid because of its higher irritant potential. Resorcinol can be found in disinfectants in concentrations at approx. 1%, which is insufficient for a peel, but is enough to disinfect surfaces.

In dermatology, resorcinol became known thanks to the American physician Max Jessner, who included it along with salicylic acid in a formulation for the hyperkeratotic epidermal lesion removal. This formulation, known as a **Jessner peel**, is used for local cauterization, while also being effective as a post-acne scar treatment, and in smoothing wrinkles and improving the overall skin tone.

1.5.1. Mechanism of action

In the Jessner peel, resorcinol is in approximately the same concentration as salicylic acid. The classic version of the Jessner peel contains the following ingredients: salicylic acid 14%, resorcinol 14%, and lactic acid 14%, with the remaining 58% comprising 95% ethanol.

How will all these substances work in the skin? Resorcinol and salicylic acid work the same way — both are keratolytic agents.

Ethanol is alcohol, a universal organic solvent that dissolves water and oil equally well. On the skin surface, ethanol quickly dissolves the hydrolipidic mantle and penetrates the intercellular spaces of the *stratum corneum*, disrupting the lipid barrier lipids. This means that salicylic acid and resorcinol more easily pass through the *stratum corneum* and get near the living cells of the epidermis faster.

Lactic acid is used to soften the effect of the two keratolytic substances and the organic solvent on the skin, but the formulation is still quite aggressive. If applied in a few layers, with increased exposure time, it results in medium-depth peeling, i.e., it causes damage at the level of the living layers of the epidermis.

1.5.2. Safety aspects

Like the salicylic peeling, Jessner peeling should not be performed on skin with sebum deficiency. The list of **contraindications** for Jessner peeling is broader than for salicylic peeling and includes the following conditions or disorders (Grimes P.E., 2006):
- Low sebum production (e.g., age-related, atopic)
- Purulent inflammatory processes in the skin
- Herpes
- Allergic reactions to peel ingredients

- Skin integrity disorders
- Pregnancy, lactation
- Thyroid dysfunction
- Diabetes mellitus
- Autoimmune diseases
- Sunburns
- Fungal skin lesions
- Keloid scars
- Couperosis
- Nevus
- During radiation and chemotherapy
- Less than two weeks after a laser or IPL treatment

1.5.3. Modified Jessner peel

Today our understanding of chemical peeling is changing — more and more practitioners prefer superficial peels that work perfectly with the *stratum corneum* and solve problems related to keratosis, fine wrinkles, spots, and uneven tone. The problems in deep layers (flabbiness, atony, microcirculation disorders) are solved by injection and physical treatments with minimal or no damage to the epidermis and skin barrier structures.

This trend is also reflected in **the modified Jessner formulas**, which successfully conquered the market because they are less traumatic. For example, resorcinol is replaced by citric or glycolic acid, and ethanol is combined with other alcohols to reduce the concentration. Here is one example of such a modification: lactic acid 17%, salicylic acid 17%, citric acid 8%, and 58% alcohol (ethanol + isopropyl alcohol). In this example, we can see another great and very modern trend: developers are looking for effective **combinations of salicylic acid with AHAs**. This is a great idea, which has significantly expanded the therapeutic possibilities of salicylic acid, which is the topic of the next chapter.

Chapter 2
Acid peels

In the mid-1990s, dermatologists turned their attention to hydroxy acids. The official recognition of these substances was preceded by a long history of their practical application. Sour milk, sugarcane juice, wine sediment, fruit, and berry juices have been used for skin rejuvenation since ancient Egypt and ancient Greece. As we already know today, some of the key active components of these products are lactic, tartaric, glycolic, and other fruit acids, which by their chemical structure belong to the hydroxy acids.

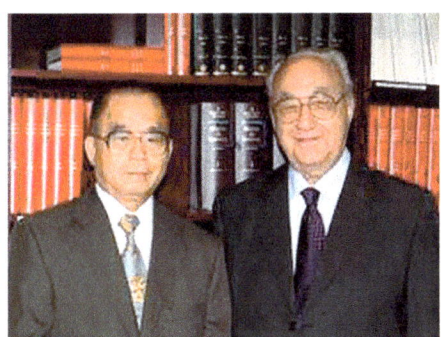

Ruey Yu and Eugene van Scott

American dermatologists Ruey Yu and Eugene van Scott were the first to study the effects of these substances on the skin in detail. Their research on hyperkeratosis conditions (e.g., ichthyosis) revealed that hydroxy acids weaken the bonds between the corneocytes, facilitating their desquamation. At the same time, unlike keratolytic agents, hydroxy acids do not denature proteins, so there is no frost on the treated area.

In addition to their exfoliating effects, hydroxy acids have been found to have other valuable properties. Today, hydroxy acids are some of the most studied and popular ingredients in topical products, which are prescribed for various skin conditions and for treating specific pathologies.

2.1. Hydroxy acids: chemical structure and classification

Organic substances containing several functional groups are called compounds with mixed functions. Such compounds include hydroxy acids having an alcohol (hydroxyl) group –OH and an acid (carboxyl) group –COOH. It turns out that a hydroxy acid is both an acid and an alcohol compound.

According to a common nomenclature variant, the carbon atom to which the carboxy group is attached is designated by the letter α, the next following atom by β, and so on, following the Greek alphabet. In the case of sufficiently long chains, the atom furthest from the carboxyl is usually designated by ω. Accordingly, if the hydroxyl group (hydroxy group) is located at the α carbon atom, the compound is called α-hydroxy acid (AHA), β-hydroxy acid (BHA) if it is found at the β atom, and so on.

The hydroxy acid molecule can contain several carboxy groups. The number of these groups is used to distinguish mono-, di-, and tricarboxylic acids. Some hydroxy acids can be classified as both AHAs and BHAs because they have a hydroxyl group in the α-position with respect to one carboxy group and in the β-position with respect to another carboxy group (**Table II-2-1**). Examples are malic and citric acids, although their chemical properties (including solubility in water) are still closer to AHAs.

There can also be a version with one carboxyl group and several hydroxyl groups. Such compounds are called polyhydroxy acids (PHAs). PHAs are widely spread and synthesized by cells from hydrocarbon compounds (including sugars) during carbohydrate metabolism reactions.

Table II-2-1. Classification of hydroxy acids (with examples)

α-HYDROXY ACIDS (AHAs)	β-HYDROXY ACIDS (BHAs)	POLYHYDROXY ACIDS (PHAs)
• Monocarboxylic: glycolic, lactic, almond • Dicarboxylic: malic, tartaric • Tricarboxylic: citric	• Propionic • β-Hydroxypropionic • Tropic	• Lactobionic • Gluconic

AHAs have a wide range of applications in skincare. These water-soluble compounds are included in emulsion and water-gel preparations, the essential characteristic of which is the pH value.

BHAs are generally less water soluble than AHAs. In addition, the mechanisms of their action, the possible positive effects on the skin, and, most importantly, the safety issues are poorly studied, so the BHAs mentioned in **Table II-2-1** are not used in cosmetics.

As for salicylic acid, it is often referred to as BHA. However, from a chemical point of view, this is incorrect because, in the salicylic acid molecule, both functional groups (carboxylic and hydroxyl) are attached directly to the benzene ring, not to the hydrocarbon chain. This fact determines salicylic acid's chemical properties and mechanism of action on the skin. Salicylic acid is insoluble in water, and its action on the skin is associated with the denaturation of proteins and does not depend on the pH value. In this respect, salicylic acid is closer to phenol and is a keratolytic agent. This point is fundamental because it explains not only the different clinical effects of salicylic acid and AHAs, but also the different approaches to developing skincare formulations and recommendations for their use. For this reason, salicylic acid is not discussed in this chapter, and information about its characteristics and use is given in Part II, section 1.4.

Two PHAs are used in dermatology and skincare: lactobionic acid and gluconic acid (and its derivative, gluconolactone). They are characterized by a pronounced moisturizing and extremely mild exfoliating effect, which makes them indispensable for the care of pathologically dry skin (ichthyosis, psoriasis).

2.2. Mechanism of action

The "leverage" of acid peeling on the skin is the change in its pH. The pH (potential of hydrogen) value is defined as the negative decimal logarithm of the concentration of hydrogen ions: pH 7 is considered neutral, pH < 7 is acidic, and pH > 7 is alkaline.

The pH value of water reflects its acid–alkaline balance, which has a significant influence on the biochemical reactions taking place in the aquatic environment. In our body, the pH value in cells and intercellular fluids is slightly alkaline and is maintained at 7.0–7.3, while in blood, the pH is slightly higher, at 7.35–7.45. But in lysosomes (the cell organelles where enzymatic digestion of macromolecules takes place), the environment is acidic: here, the concentration of hydrogen ions is more than 100 times higher than in the cytoplasm, so the pH is within the 4.5–5.5 range.

As no living cells exist in the *stratum corneum*, the pH situation is quite different. Across the *stratum corneum*, the pH changes gradually from an acidic 4.6–5.5 in the hydrolipid mantle to a slightly alkaline 7 at the border with the granular layer. This is an extreme pH difference, and it occurs within the thin *stratum corneum*. **Fig. II-2-1** shows how the pH changes within the *stratum corneum*.

The pH gradient is a key factor in regulating enzymatic activity within the *stratum corneum*, which is quite variable. Proteolytic enzymes (closer to the surface) cleave corneodesmosomes and induce corneocyte exfoliation. In the lower layers of the *stratum corneum*, other enzymes are active: some are responsible for transforming keratinocytes into corneocytes, and others for forming intercellular lipid structures comprising the lipid barrier.

All enzymes have their pH optimum: some are more active in an acidic environment, others in a more alkaline one. A pH deviation from the optimum inevitably affects the enzymatic activity: it decreases gradually and eventually ceases completely.

If a preparation with a pH that differs significantly from 5.5 is applied to the skin surface, the surface pH value and the pH gradient through the *stratum corneum* change. This disrupts the physiological conditions required by the enzymes of the *stratum corneum* to work optimally. During natural epidermis renewal, the defective horny scales reach the surface and peel off in a few days. Ordinarily, we do not see scaling because the normal horny scales are too small. In contrast, after acid peeling, the flaking is visible as larger abnormal horny scales formed due to the rapid change in pH are leaving the skin.

In addition to enzyme failure, the pH change affects the structures maintaining the integrity of the *stratum corneum*, namely:
- Intercellular lipid layers that "glue" corneocytes
- Corneodesmosomes which are protein bridges between neighboring corneocytes, ensuring their adhesion to each other

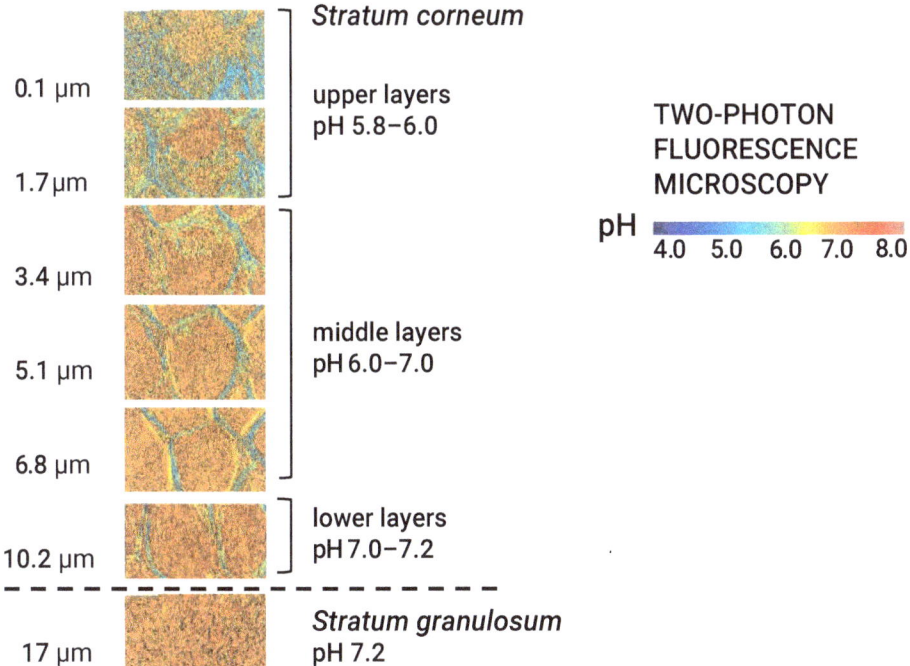

Figure II-2-1. pH gradient through the *stratum corneum*: measurements by two-photon fluorescence microscopy (Hanson K.M. et al., 2002)

Special molecules — fluorescent probes — are applied to the skin. They penetrate the *stratum corneum* and, under subsequent irradiation with light of a specific wavelength, go into an excited state and then give off excess energy in the form of photons (quanta of light). This secondary radiation is called fluorescence and can be recorded. To determine the pH of the *stratum corneum*, a probe was chosen that can emit in both acidic and alkaline environments, but this emission is at different wavelengths. The resulting image indicates the luminescence in the acidic environment in blue and the neutral–alkaline environment in orange. These colored images can thus be used to calculate the average pH at different depths of the *stratum corneum* as the ratio of the blue areas to the orange areas.

It is evident from the image above that blue color is more present closer to the surface. The calculated average pH value in the upper *stratum corneum* layers is slightly higher than in the hydrolipid mantle but still acidic — less than 7. In the middle of the *stratum corneum*, the pH is close to neutral. At the very depth, it becomes slightly alkaline.

The distribution of color in the *stratum corneum* is uneven. Blue (acidic) areas are separated from orange (neutral) areas. The *stratum corneum* consists of dense, almost waterless corneocytes, and inside them, pH is neutral. Free water in the *stratum corneum* is present in the intercellular space, and this water, as clearly shown here, will be acidified. That is, even in the lowest layers of the *stratum corneum*, we still see areas with acidic pH, although there are fewer of them.

Under the *stratum corneum*, water is everywhere — both in the cells and in the intercellular space. The pH here is slightly alkaline, so we don't see individual cells, but rather uniform orange staining.

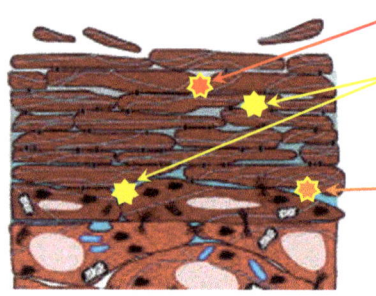

- Corneodesmosomes
- Enzymes of the *stratum corneum* (proteolytic enzymes, enzymes assembling the lipid barrier)
- Intracellular lipid lamellar structures

Figure II-2-2. Acid peel targets

These structures contain molecules with charged groups giving rise to electrostatic interactions. These interactions weaken as the pH environment changes, making the *stratum corneum* looser and less strong.

Thus, the change in pH gradient through the *stratum corneum* "hits" three key points controlling the formation and integrity of the skin barrier (**Fig. II-2-2**):
1. *Stratum corneum*'s enzymes
2. Intercellular lipid layers
3. Corneodesmosomes

It should be noted that the pH gradient through the *stratum corneum* changes when both acidic and alkaline substances are applied to the skin. In both cases, the skin peels as a result. So, alkaline preparations can also be used if our goal is to cause flaking. Remember how skin peels after washing with laundry soap? That's because the soap solution has an alkaline pH of 9–11. Yet, alkaline peels are considered exotic today, but acidic peels are widespread and are successfully used in different situations. In terms of safety, acidifying the surface pH is much better tolerated by the skin and is safer than alkalizing it.

The more the pH gradient changes and the longer this condition lasts, the stronger the exfoliation. Therefore, the power of the acid peel depends on the formulation's pH and exposure time.
The acid concentration is not critical: for example, a formulation with a total AHA concentration of up to 70% and a pH of 5.5 does not exfoliate. On the contrary, a product with 30% AHA content and a pH 1.5 causes noticeable scaling.

The burning sensation that appears some time after applying acid peels indicates that the acidification has progressed beyond the *stratum corneum*. Nerve endings, distributed in the skin in high density, communicate with all skin cells — mast cells, endothelial cells, keratinocytes, Langerhans cells, and fibroblasts. In response to an external stimulus (e.g., a decrease in the pH of the intercellular space), nerve endings release neuropeptides such as the substance P (SP) or calcitonin gene-related peptide (CGRP) acting on neighboring cells. In turn, the cells release histamine and pro-inflammatory cytokines, which activate sensory nerve endings and trigger a signal transmission to the brain — this is the signal we perceive as burning. Histamine dilates blood vessels and provides blood flow to the problematic area to dissolve and eliminate irritants as quickly as possible (Choi J.E., Di Nardo A., 2018). If the acid action is not stopped, an inflammatory reaction (so-called **neurogenic inflammation**) is triggered in the epidermis (**Fig. II-2-3**).

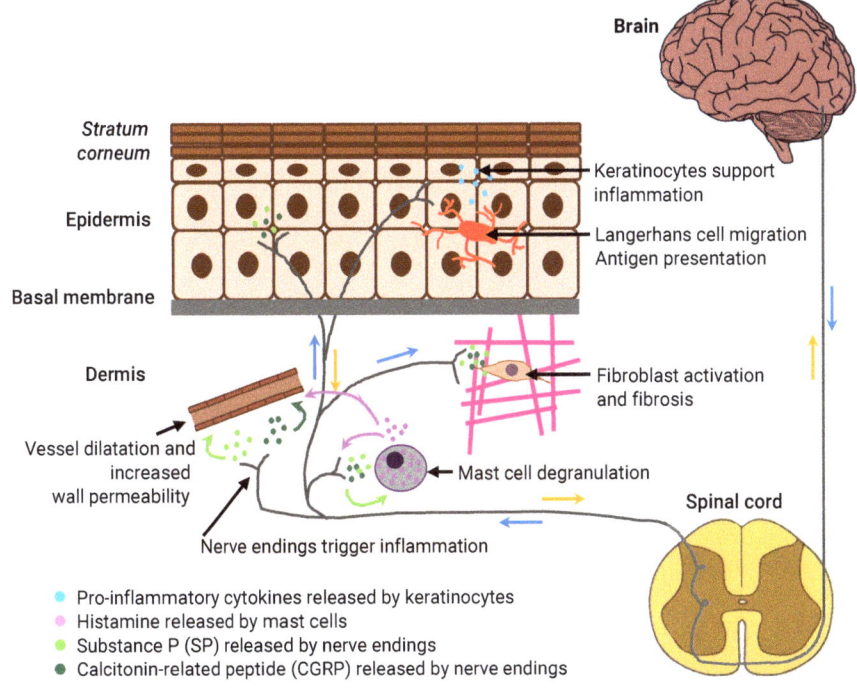

Figure II-2-3. Neurogenic inflammation in the skin (Choi J.E., Di Nardo A., 2018)

The question of whether it is necessary to provoke an inflammatory response remains open because the primary goal of chemical peel — exfoliation — can be achieved without it. Some practitioners believe that inflammation is appropriate if, in addition to exfoliation, we want to activate remodeling processes in the dermis. This activation is indirect and is triggered by mediators released by epidermal cells. Other practitioners prefer more effective and comfortable minimally invasive injections or physical treatments for remodeling, and perform chemical peel for light exfoliation.

You can stop the acid peel action at any time with the help of a neutralizer. A neutralizer is an alkaline solution in which sodium bicarbonate is usually the main active ingredient. Additionally, it can include moisturizing and softening agents such as β-glucan, plant extracts, and free amino acids.

2.3. α-Hydroxy acids (AHAs)

AHAs are often referred to as fruit acids because they are found in many fruits. Skincare products containing fruit acids were first launched in the early 1990s and quickly gained popularity due to the rapidity of results. However, the euphoria was short-lived. The increasing complaints of skin irritation and even burns lowered the rating of AHA-containing cosmetics and made scientists take the problem of their creation and application seriously. As a result of numerous studies, they established the optimal parameters for ensuring that skincare products with AHAs are effective and safe.

2.3.1. AHAs for topical application

The AHAs used as cosmetic ingredients are discussed next.

Glycolic acid

Glycolic acid is the simplest hydroxy acid. It is found in sugarcane and green grapes.

Glycolic acid has the lowest molecular weight among the AHAs, so it penetrates the epidermal barrier faster than the others. Glycolic acid is most often used in acid peel formulations where its concentration can be up to 70%. Still, as we have already mentioned, it is not the concentration that determines the intensity of exfoliation, but the pH value, which can be adjusted to the desired level with any acid concentration.

Glycolic acid has other valuable properties, but they manifest at low concentrations (about 1–2%). Thus, treatment with a 2% glycolic acid solution increases skin resistance to UV light and can be considered a prevention of photoaging. The subtle mechanisms of this effect are under investigation, but it is already known that UV-induced processes develop less intensively in the skin prepared in this way. UV exposure suppresses the expression of aquaporin-3 (a transmembrane protein that forms the channel for the transport of water and osmolytes into the cell and is involved in the regulation of water balance in the living skin layers) and increases the activity of matrix metalloproteinases that degrade collagen, resulting in clinical manifestations of photoaging such as skin dehydration and early wrinkles. These processes are less pronounced in the skin treated with glycolic acid preparations (Tang S.-C. et al., 2019). In addition, the skin treated with 2% glycolic acid has a reduced level of reactive oxygen species (ROS) and pro-inflammatory mediators after UV irradiation, so erythema is less pronounced than in the untreated skin (Hung S.J. et al., 2017; Tang S.-C., Yang J.-H., 2018).

Lactic acid

Lactic acid is a monobasic carboxylic acid with three carbon atoms containing a hydroxyl group. Salts and esters of lactic acid are called lactates. Lactic acid is formed by the lactic fermentation of sugars and plays an essential role in metabolism.

Lactic acid was first isolated in 1780. L-lactic acid is produced by the lactic acid bacteria *Lactobacillus* and is responsible for the smell of fermented milk. D-lactic acid, also called sarcolactic acid, is produced by anaerobic muscle contraction. In nature, D-lactic acid is found in apples, ergot, foxglove, opium, tomatoes, blueberries, passionflower, maple syrup, and grapes.

It is part of the *stratum corneum*'s natural moisturizing factor (NMF). It has a pronounced hydrating and mild exfoliating effect on the skin, so it is often used in moisturizing care products. It is included in peel formulations to reduce irritation and soften the peel's effect on the skin (for example, Jessner peel, see Part II, section 1.5). It is especially recommended for baby skin and dry skin of the elderly. In these life periods, there is a physiological deficiency of NMF, so applying the cream containing lactic acid, ceramides, and squalene greatly helps and provides prolonged hydration.

Pyruvic acid

Pyruvic acid is an α-keto analog of lactic acid formed in cells during the pyrolysis of tartaric acid. It plays an important role in cell metabolism, acting as a "crossroads" of many metabolic pathways, particularly in glucose metabolism.

Topical pyruvic acid has keratolytic, bactericidal, and sebostatic properties, so it is used for treating acne, superficial scars, photodamage, and pigmentation disorders.

A peel formulation with pyruvic acid as the main active ingredient is known as Red Peel. Red Peel is designed for superficial and medium-depth peels containing no more than 50% of pyruvic acid in their composition.

Applying pyruvic acid causes an intense burning sensation; erythema and intense scaling (up to crusting) develop a little later. To reduce the discomfort and the risk of adverse reactions, antioxidant and moisturizing components are added to the formulations. Thus, modern preparations are milder than pure pyruvic acid solutions with similar pyruvic acid concentrations.

A comparison of pyruvic acid peels (50%) and salicylic acid peels (30%) in the treatment of mild to moderate acne showed no differences in therapeutic and adverse effects (Jaffary F. et al., 2016). When pyruvic acid peel (50%) was compared to a peel containing glycolic and salicylic acids, their therapeutic effectiveness in the treatment of acne was also comparable. However, in terms of tolerability of the procedure and adverse reactions such as burning sensation, erythema, and edema, the complex peel is milder (Zdrada J. et al., 2020).

Mandelic acid

Mandelic acid is the first representative of aromatic hydroxy acids with an aliphatic chain. It is a colorless crystalline solid substance that is slightly soluble in water and well-soluble in polar organic solvents — in alcohols and diethyl ether. Mandelic acid is obtained by hydrolysis of bitter almond extract.

On the skin, mandelic acid acts quite mildly, so it is used in combination with other AHAs in peel formulations and moisturizers for routine skincare (Yevglevskis M. et al., 2014).

Tartaric acid

Tartaric acid is a dibasic oxyacid. Widely distributed in the plant world, it occurs as free isomers and acidic salts. Its primary source is mature grapes. The substance is released during the fermentation of berry juice, forming hard-to-dissolve potassium salts called tartrate. The food additive is registered under code E334 and is obtained from secondary wine processing products (yeast, chalky sediment, tartaric lime).

When applied to the skin, tartaric acid has an exfoliating, whitening, moisturizing, and antioxidant effect. It is found in peel formulas and skincare products intended for treating uneven pigmentation and signs of photoaging.

Malic acid

Malic acid is a dibasic keto acid. This intermediate product of the tricarboxylic acid and glyoxylate cycles was first isolated from unripe apples in 1785. It is found in many fruits, especially apples, grapes, rowanberries, etc.

Malic acid has antioxidant, cleansing, moisturizing, anti-inflammatory, and slightly astringent properties. In addition to exfoliating, it activates metabolic processes in living cells. It is found in superficial acid peels. Some studies show a positive effect of malic acid on the skin in atopic dermatitis (Tang S.-C., Yang J.-H., 2018; Lee B. et al., 2019).

Citric acid

Citric acid is a tribasic carboxylic acid. It is found in various fruits, but its quantities are particularly large in citrus fruits (up to about 5% in fruit and up to 9% in juice). Citric acid is involved in the tricarboxylic acid cycle — the main process of cell respiration. Accordingly, it is found in all animals and plants in appreciable concentrations.

Citric acid has higher molecular weight than the AHAs discussed above. In cosmetic products, it is most often used as a pH regulator. In addition to this technical function, citric acid also has biological properties: it lightens the skin (especially in the presence of tartaric acid) and has antioxidant and bactericidal effects.

2.3.2. Clinical effects

The clinical effects of AHAs on the skin can be divided into two groups:
1. **Non-specific effects** typical of all AHAs — determined by the pH of the finished product and consist of accelerating desquamation and epidermal cell turnover, which is clinically expressed in the special skin scaling
2. **Specific effects** related to the chemical characteristics and concentration of a particular AHA which are based on the specific target effect on the skin

The expression and predominance of one or another effect in the clinical picture depends on the peel formulation features and the skin's initial state. The components that determine the total effect are discussed in detail in the following sections.

Scaling

This is the main effect of acid peeling. Unlike keratolytic agents, the scaling effect of which is manifested already during the procedure in the form of frost, fine flaking of the skin after acid peeling becomes noticeable in a few days (usually on the 2nd–3rd day) and lasts for several days. This delay is due to the peculiarities of the mechanism of action based on a sharp shift of the pH gradient through the *stratum corneum* (see Part II, section 2.2).

Moisturizing

As corneocytes move toward the surface, the NMF components degrade, and the corneocytes become drier, stiffer, and more brittle. The rapid shedding of the *stratum corneum* flakes and the renewal of the epidermis leads to an increase in the content of functionally active NMF and, consequently, the water associated with it. Thus, the renewal of the *stratum corneum* itself has a positive effect on its hydration.

In addition, lactic acid (one of the AHAs) is also one of the NMF components. It is hygroscopic and retains water molecules through electrostatic interactions. Lactic acid is found in sweat and is excreted with it to the skin surface. It is further reabsorbed and accumulated in the *stratum corneum*, maintaining the pH gradient and the hydration level.

Soothing

Strange as it may seem, AHA-containing formulations may exhibit anti-inflammatory properties, reducing superoxide and hydroxyl radical production and modulating the functional activity of B- and T-lymphocytes. However, this effect is related to the products with a relatively low AHA concentration and a pH above 3.5.

The AHAs' anti-inflammatory effects are expressed in different degrees and are directly related to their respective antioxidant properties. Thus, a comparison of three AHAs (glycolic, lactic, and tartaric) and one PHA (gluconolactone) showed that tartaric acid and gluconolactone, which are also more potent antioxidants, have a more effective anti-inflammatory effect (Berardesca E. et al., 1997).

Still, the antioxidant properties of the AHAs are not very pronounced. When AHAs are combined with other antioxidants, a synergistic effect can appear, and the antioxidant potential of the composition increases significantly. The role of AHAs, in this case, is a reduction of the second component, increasing the overall antioxidant potential.

2.3.3. Features of AHA-containing formulations

The clinical effect severity depends mainly on how much of the active substance reaches its target. The fact is that, once in the skin, AHAs are distributed unevenly and can selectively accumulate in certain areas. Penetration can be enhanced by introducing several substances into the formulation, such as glycols. Penetration depends on the pH: it decreases with increasing pH and becomes minimal at pH 7.

This dependence is very important because the irritant potential of AHA-containing products is related to the pH value. Around pH 3.5, their irritant potential decreases sharply. Comparison of these data with the penetration depths allowed us to determine the optimal pH value (3.5–4.0) at which the product is effective and relatively safe.

The division of AHA products into cosmetic and medical is somewhat arbitrary. Cosmetic products can be bought without a prescription and used at home, and medical products are used under the supervision of a professional in an outpatient setting. According to the U.S. Food and Drug Administration (FDA), the first category includes products with no more than 10% AHA and a pH of at least 3.5. The second category includes products with more than 10% AHA and a pH below 3.5. Products with 30–40% AHA are allowed in the aesthetic practice. Preparations with 50–70% AHA and a pH of about 1.0 are permitted for use only by medical professionals.

Let us focus on some important points that must be considered by cosmetics manufacturers that develop and produce finished products and by aestheticians who use them in their practice.

Combinations of active ingredients

Despite the variety of AHAs, glycolic acid remains the main component of acid peels. The other AHAs are also found in peel products but are usually combined with glycolic acid. In at-home and pre-peel products, their peeling effect is less strong, but they have some specific characteristics, such as whitening and moisturizing. That is why AHAs are desirable ingredients for aging skin, skin damaged by UV rays, oily skin prone to blackheads, and even dry skin.

Often AHAs are combined with salicylic acid. Such combined preparations are emulsions — they have both an aqueous phase where the AHAs are localized and an oil phase where salicylic acid is concentrated. The addition of AHAs allows for a lower concentration of salicylic acid while maintaining the overall exfoliating power. Such preparations can be used even on sebum-deficient skin (which, remember, is a contraindication for using salicylic acid, see Part II, section 1.3.2).

AHA formulations often include antioxidants (e.g., vitamins C and E) and plant extracts with a variety of properties (anti-inflammatory, moisturizing, and sedative) (Taylor M.B. et al., 2013). Formulations developed for pigmented skin include bleaching agents such as arbutin or kojic acid. AHA products also contain biologically active components such as hyaluronic acid, pyroglutamic acid, squalene, peptides and amino acids, urea, and phytoestrogens, the effectiveness of which increases in the presence of AHA. This is understandable because AHA increases the barrier's permeability and facilitates the passage of other components through it.

In several studies on the combined action of AHAs with estrogens, the simultaneous use of a cream with glycolic acid and a cream with estradiol was shown to result in a slightly more pronounced increase in epidermal thickness. In skincare practice, estrogens are prohibited, but there are formulations where AHAs are combined with substances of plant origin that have an estrogen-like effect on the skin (phytoestrogens) (Fuchs K.O. et al., 2003).

Optimal base

The medium in which AHAs are found plays an important role in the final efficacy of cosmetic and dermatological preparations. Since most AHAs are water-soluble, they are preferably placed in aqueous gels or in creams and lotions that are oil-in-water emulsions. Some AHAs (e.g., almond oil) are quite soluble in the oil phase, so that preparations can be created as water-in-oil emulsions or as ointments. The occlusive properties of such preparations contribute to the AHA penetration.

The goals of the formulators also determine the choice of medium for AHAs. Some specific skin conditions, such as severe dryness, may require water-soluble AHAs. Hence, the AHA product should be an oil-in-water emulsion so that the AHA molecules accumulate in a continuous external aqueous phase, become more bioavailable for the skin, and fulfill their therapeutic purpose. After just a few days of topical application of such products, dry skin scaling is significantly reduced since the acids activate the natural desquamation mechanisms (the ties between the scales are loosened, and they wash away during a bath or a shower). On the contrary, the effectiveness of glycolic acid decreases dramatically if the product containing it is a water-in-oil emulsion.

For eczematous skin, the preferred form of preparations is a water-in-oil ointment or emulsion containing small amounts of mild AHAs (lactic acid is the best option) and having a pH of about 5.0–5.6, which would not irritate sensitive or inflamed skin. In psoriasis, the most beneficial effect can be obtained if the formulations include occlusive components, such as petroleum jelly (a mixture of paraffin, petroleum oil, and ceresin) or mineral oil.

Other base substances can also influence the AHA effectiveness. For example, glycerin — a moisturizer in many cosmetic products — has a high affinity to water-soluble AHAs. Since glycerin does not penetrate well through the *stratum corneum*, its simultaneous application to the skin surface reduces the penetration ability of AHAs and thus weakens their local effects (except for moisturizing). Other excipients can, on the contrary, intensify the AHA effects. For example, propylene glycol increases the permeability of the *stratum corneum* and facilitates AHA penetration into the skin.

pH of the finished product

The dilemma for the formulators is to increase the active ingredient concentration as much as possible but to avoid the irritation associated with low pH. This is especially true in the case of very dry skin with compromised barrier properties. The solution is to neutralize the formulation, for which sodium bicarbonate (baking soda) is traditionally used.

Yu R.J. and van Scott E.J. (2002) suggested using amphoteric amino acids — arginine, lysine, glycine — as neutralizing agents. Free amino acids are primarily moisturizing agents that are natural for the *stratum corneum* because they are part of the NMF. The amphoteric ingredients form complexes with the AHAs, which break down over time, gradually releasing their components. Thus, the problems of low pH and moisturizing the dry *stratum corneum* are solved simultaneously.

2.3.4. Indications and practical aspects

Skincare routine, age-related changes prevention, and treatment

In skincare practice, it is not uncommon to use a complex of several acids with complementary action. AHAs are combined with other bioactive substances (see above) in products for specific applications. The main indications for using AHA-based products for cosmetic purposes are presented in **Table II-2-2**.

Table II-2-2. Indications for the use of cosmetic products with AHAs

SKIN CONDITION	MECHANISM OF ACTION AND CLINICAL EFFECTS
Dry skin	The total moisture content of the *stratum corneum* is increased by strengthening its water-holding and water-regulating systems: • Removal of old corneocytes from the surface promotes faster renewal of the cellular composition while also strengthening the barrier function of the epidermis (TEWL decreases, NMF increases) • Stimulation of restoration of intercellular lipid layers of the *stratum corneum*
Oily skin prone to blackheads	• Reducing the cohesion of corneocytes facilitates the clearing of blocked sebaceous gland ducts • Exfoliation opens the sebaceous ducts and makes sebaceous glands accessible to biologically active components that reduce sebum formation, normalize lipid metabolism, and have a bactericidal effect • Reducing the likelihood of scarring in acne disease • Prevention and treatment of hyperpigmentation that can occur with acne disease
Fading skin	• Renewing the epidermal cellular composition of the skin by exfoliating and proliferating basal keratinocytes • Facilitating penetration into the deeper layers of the skin of other active ingredients in the formulation • Moisturizing effect • Smoothing the skin by increasing its hydration and stimulating the synthesis of collagen and glycosaminoglycans
Pigmented skin	• Facilitating the penetration of bleaching agents into the skin • Direct bleaching effect of some AHAs (e.g., tartaric and citric acid)

Abbreviations: TEWL — transepidermal water loss; NMF — natural moisturizing factor

AHA preparations are developed with different skin types in mind. Emulsion formulations (creams, lotions) are better suited for individuals with dry skin, as well as older patients with pigmented skin. Lotions, which may contain mild surfactants, are recommended for younger patients with oily skin and comedones.

Cosmetic products with up to 10% AHA in their composition are widely used at the stage of skin preparation for chemical peeling. The result of their application is a thinning of the *stratum corneum*, which allows the peel procedure to be better tolerated in the future and ensures more even and rapid penetration of the active ingredients through the barrier.

In the early post-peel period, when the skin barrier has not fully recovered, it is better not to use products with AHAs, as they can traumatize the skin even in small concentrations. Afterward, when the barrier function has been restored, such preparations can be used for short-term supportive and preventive care, and then you have to take a break.

Initially, low AHA concentrations are advised, with gradual increases, while carefully observing the tolerability of the drug. The skin should be closely monitored, and the drug should be discontinued immediately at the first sign of discomfort or visible adverse reaction (mild rash, redness).

Acne, post-acne

In acne, the weakening of adhesion of corneocytes and loosening of the *stratum corneum* near the mouths of the follicles makes it easier to squeeze out comedones and prevents their recurrence.

As an outpatient, a 50–70% aqueous solution of glycolic acid can be used to treat the affected skin area with a cotton swab. After a few minutes, redness appears, and a slight swelling develops around the follicles. As soon as the first symptoms of erythema appear, the skin should be washed thoroughly with a neutralizer. After such treatment, comedones are much easier to remove, even from hard-to-reach areas.

Preparations with low AHA concentrations, containing water, propylene glycol, and a small ethanol concentration, can be used for preventive skin cleansing. Their regular use precludes follicle re-clogging.

In addition, they acidify the skin, which is important for restoring the acid mantle (acne is known to alkalize the skin surface).

In the case of post-acne scars and enlarged pores, an acid peeling will not alleviate these issues, but it will smooth out the microrelief and lighten the blemishes to a degree, so that the skin looks fresher and has healthier appearance.

Atopic dermatitis

In atopic dermatitis, as in acne, the surface pH increases to 6.5, which disturbs the microbiome. Therefore, regular use of acidifying agents with AHAs is indicated for such skin. It is best to use lactic acid, which additionally moisturizes the skin. The care product should have a pH of 4.0–4.5 and should contain special buffering substances that maintain this pH level after application on the skin.

In the remission stage, light acid peeling can be performed if there are no contraindications. The pH of the peel should be at 3.0–3.5, and the AHA concentration should not exceed 20%.

Pseudofolliculitis barbae

Pseudofolliculitis barbae is an inflammatory reaction around ingrown hairs that occurs after shaving. People with curly hair often encounter this problem. More than 50% of black men suffer to a greater or lesser extent from pustules appearing on their faces after shaving. Women are also affected, and pustules can occur after shaving their legs and pubic area, where hair is particularly stiff.

Pseudofolliculitis barbae is characteristic of curly hair that bends as it grows. When a curly hair leaves the follicle, it can penetrate the epidermis, forming an ingrown hair. When shaving obliquely, the cut hair leaves a fairly sharp end that easily pierces the epidermis. A stiff, wavy hair can also penetrate the epidermis without leaving the follicle, as is often the case when shaving with a razor blade. Once the free end of the hair penetrates the epidermis, inflammation and intraepidermal microabscess begin. The hair continues to grow and reaches the dermis, where *pseudofolliculitis barbae* — an abscess involving immune cells (macrophages, lymphocytes) develops around the hair.

Regular use of AHA lotions has proven effective for this problem. However, in this situation, the AHA action is based on a different mechanism from that previously described. As AHAs are reducing agents by their chemical nature, it is very likely that they can repair the sulfur-containing groups by breaking the sulfhydryl bonds (the number of which determines the degree of hair curliness) and straightening the hair. The risk of *pseudofolliculitis barbae* is reduced because straight hair is less likely to ingrow into the epidermis than curly hair. To prevent *pseudofolliculitis barbae*, buffered lotions containing 8% glycolic acid are recommended. Their daily use makes life much easier for curly-haired men and women who use razors for hair removal.

Ichthyosis

This pathology is characterized by a thickened *stratum corneum*. Lotions, gels, and creams with a pH of 3.5–4.0 and up to 12% AHA content are suitable for prevention and treatment. Regular daily use of these products for lamellar ichthyosis may be even more effective than systemic therapy with retinoids. Glycolic and lactic acids or their derivatives are most often used. But polyhydroxy acids have proven even more effective (see below).

Keratosis

Before any form of keratosis can be treated, an accurate diagnosis must be made to rule out malignant skin growth. Therefore, treatment should begin with a visit to a physician, who will diagnose and prescribe an appropriate course of therapy.

The main sign of keratosis is hyperkeratinization, which is a local pathological thickening of the epidermis, especially its *stratum corneum*. Hyperkeratinization may be accompanied by hyperpigmentation, so the thickened areas often look darker compared to the normal skin color.

One of the most common manifestations of keratosis is age spots (lentigines). These thickened brown formations vary in size and shade (from light to dark). Patients usually complain of age spots on the face and hands, which is a severe cosmetic disadvantage. The spots can be removed with a concentrated solution of AHA, which causes epidermolysis — complete disaggregation of keratinocytes and breaking of dermo-epidermal bonds. The treated area of the epidermis is then easily removed to the level of the basal membrane by gentle scraping. The strongest remedy for removing age spots is a formulation of

100% pyruvic acid, which is liquid at room temperature. First, the skin is degreased with 70% ethanol solution, then 1–2 drops of the preparation are applied to the affected area without preliminary anesthesia. A thin camel hair brush is used for precise application.

In the case of squamous keratoses on the face, epidermolysis usually occurs within one minute. As soon as the epidermis in the treated area becomes loose, it should be scraped off immediately. Then the skin should be rinsed thoroughly with water to remove the remaining acid and prevent further penetration. If this is not done, deeper penetration can later lead to the development of persistent erythema and the formation of an undesirable crust. The same procedure can also be used to remove solar keratoses and lentigines.

Less concentrated solutions — 50% pyruvic acid in aqueous–alcoholic solution, as well as aqueous solutions of glycolic acid (70%) and lactic acid (85%), can be used to induce delayed epidermolysis in lesions on large areas.

After re-epithelialization, which lasts several days depending on the area and site of treatment, erythema remains for 2–3 weeks. The treated skin looks much smoother than the surrounding areas. This condition can last for weeks or even months.

Removal of keratoses with concentrated solutions should be performed on an outpatient basis. Less concentrated preparations can be used at home and are quite effective in the initial stages. The best results are achieved with creams, lotions, and gels with 10–12% AHA partially neutralized by ammonium salts. To achieve visible results, they should be used regularly, strictly following the instructions. The time it takes to achieve a clinical effect range from a few weeks to 9–12 months.

A daily application of AHA preparation gradually loosens and thins the *stratum corneum*. Additional skin lightening can be achieved by adding bleaching agents such as kojic acid and arbutin. In the typical case of localized spots on the hands, patients can apply alcohol and water–alcoholic solutions of 20% glycolic acid directly to the spots with a special brush. Subsequent application of a cosmetic cream, lotion, or gel with AHA accelerates the appearance of the desired results.

In the case of solar keratoses, doctors recommend combining the drug 5-fluorouracil with AHA therapy. This shortens the treatment duration and alleviates the feeling of discomfort.

Warts

The fight against warts of viral nature is conducted on two fronts:
1. Destruction
2. Disruption of virus replication

The wart tissue can be destroyed with epidermolysis-inducing AHAs, while the virus lifecycle is disrupted with an appropriate drug, such as 5-fluorouracil. Of course, epidermolysis can also be used to remove the wart by pulling it out by the root, but clinical experience shows that the best results are achieved with a combination of AHA therapy and 5-fluorouracil.

For outpatient procedures, a 1–2% solution of 5-fluorouracil in glycolic or pyruvic acid is typically prepared. After the wart is trimmed, a piece of absorbent cotton soaked in the solution is placed on it and fixed with a plaster. After a few hours, the patient removes the application. One procedure is sufficient in the case of relatively mild warts on the face. For warts on the palms or soles, it is usually necessary to repeat the procedure several times.

Less concentrated solutions are used at home — 0.5% 5-fluorouracil in an alcoholic solution of AHAs (AHAs/ethanol in a 1:1 ratio).

2.3.5. Contraindications and safety

Without exception, patients with thin, non-greasy skin and minimal pigmentation are more sensitive to AHAs than patients with oily and pigmented skin. General advice for those considering the use of AHAs: start with low concentrations and gradually move up to higher ones, carefully observing the patient's tolerance of the product. Sometimes irritation does not occur immediately but after prolonged use. In this case, either temporal or permanent cessation is necessary.

Contraindications to the use AHA-containing topical products are:
- Individual intolerance
- Skin hypersensitivity
- Injured skin
- Herpetic rashes

- Telangiectasias
- Prolonged sun exposure

Adherence to the following **basic safety precautions** is advised when using topical products with AHAs:
1. Always protect your skin before going outdoors. Use sunscreen with an SPF of 15 or higher. Wear a hat and clothing that covers treated skin areas.
2. Use only preparations that contain all the necessary information: (1) complete list of ingredients; (2) AHA concentration; (3) pH; (4) name of the manufacturing company and address of that company or its distributor. The first three items are mandatory; the fourth is optional.
3. Before using the drug, you should perform a control test — apply a small amount of the drug on the back of your hand and watch the reaction overnight.
4. Discontinue use immediately if signs of an adverse reaction appear. These signs include burning, redness, itching, tingling, pain, bleeding, and increased sensitivity to sunlight.

Adhering to these measures is not difficult, but they will preclude serious problems that can arise from a seemingly innocuous and promising cosmetic product.

> After acid peeling and against the background of the application of skincare cosmetics with AHAs, the skin becomes more even and luminous. The overall clinical result is due to the multiple biological effects of AHAs. They activate cell renewal in the epidermis, reducing the *stratum corneum* thickness and increasing its hydration; due to the exfoliation, they reduce the amount of melanin in the epidermis and lighten the skin. The anti-inflammatory effect of AHAs is attributed to their antioxidant properties and ability to influence inflammatory mediators' release. With long-term use of skincare products with AHAs, a slight lifting may be observed in some cases due to an improvement in the quality of the dermal matrix, but this effect is associated with an indirect effect on fibroblasts through cytokines that release epidermal cells in response to AHAs.

2.4. Polyhydroxy acids (PHAs)

How to preserve the beneficial properties of AHAs but avoid burning? Many pharmaceutical and cosmetic companies are working in this direction. One elegant and productive solution was proposed by Yu R.J. and van Scott E.J. (2002). They pointed out that polyhydroxy acids are better tolerated by the skin and moisturize it better than glycolic acid, commonly used as a peeling agent. Several PHAs were identified as a result of their research and are briefly discussed below.

2.4.1. Lactobionic acid

Lactobionic acid is a 4-O-β-D-galactopyranosyl-D-gluconic acid consisting of gluconic acid and galactose. It may be formed during the oxidation of disaccharide lactose. It forms salts with metals such as calcium, potassium, sodium, and zinc.

Lactobionic acid is a hybrid consisting of galactose sugar and gluconic acid (according to the classification, it belongs to the class of bionic polyhydroxy acids). A molecule of lactobionic acid has eight hydroxyl groups, which means that it can "bind" eight water molecules to itself by ionic bonds (for comparison, gluconolactone has four hydroxyl groups, lactic and glycolic acids have one each). Therefore, lactobionic acid is an excellent moisturizer, acting in a similar way to the components of the natural moisturizing factor, i.e., concentrating in the *stratum corneum* and attracting water to itself. Moreover, its water-absorbing and water-holding properties are superior to most hygroscopic compounds typically used in topical preparations (Tasić-Kostov M. et al., 2019).

The safety of lactobionic acid is confirmed by the fact that it is used in the food industry and pharmacy (usually in salt form). For example, calcium lactobionate is used in the food industry as a stabilizer.

Potassium lactobionate is added to special solutions designed for the osmotic stabilization of cells and tissues. The mineral salts of lactobionate are used as mineral food additives. When administered intravenously, the antibiotic erythromycin is used in salt form (erythromycin lactobionate). Experiments have also revealed a positive effect of lactobionic acid on the dermal matrix. It is assumed that it inhibits matrix metalloproteinases, slowing down the destruction of collagen and elastin. After long-term use of preparations with lactobionic acid, the biomechanical properties of the skin, including elasticity and tensile strength, improve.

All these qualities make lactobionic acid a valuable ingredient in topical preparations designed for:
- Deep and lasting hydration (aimed at dry and very dry skin, skin with damaged *stratum corneum*, photodamaged skin)
- Restorative care after aesthetic procedures (such as microdermabrasion, chemical peeling, non-ablative phototherapy, mesotherapy)

In addition to their moisturizing effect, PHAs loosen the *stratum corneum*, accelerating the renewal of the epidermal cellular composition. Both properties are particularly useful for ichthyosis where timely removal of keratinized masses and deep moisturizing needs to be achieved simultaneously.

2.4.2. Gluconic acid and gluconolactone

Gluconic acid ($C_6H_{12}O_7$) is an organic acid of the aldonic acid group. It is formed by the oxidation of the aldehyde group of glucose. The phosphorylated form of gluconic acid is an important intermediate product of carbohydrate metabolism in living cells. The compound activates metabolism in the body, increases muscle performance, and has other beneficial effects on the body.

Both gluconic acid and its derivative gluconolactone are used in skincare practice. Both compounds have good moisturizing and mild keratolytic effects, an optimal combination for very dry and sensitive skin. They also have antioxidant properties, which are also helpful for seriously compromised skin barrier and defense systems. Ichthyosis patients have insufficient protease activity of the *stratum corneum*, which results in impaired desquamation.

PHAs do not increase the skin sensitivity to sunlight and can be used as a part of a comprehensive treatment program that includes retinoids and other cosmetic products. Since the molecules of these substances are larger than those of AHAs, they penetrate much more slowly, allowing them to accumulate within the *stratum corneum*. This is a big advantage because the task of the PHAs is to act on the *stratum corneum*, not on living cells.

Gluconolactone is a lactone (cyclic ester) of D-gluconic acid. It is obtained by bacterial fermentation of pure glucose to form gluconic acid and subsequent evaporation of the solution. It is a white crystalline powder with a faint characteristic odor. It is soluble in water and glycerin, insoluble in ethyl alcohol and vegetable oil.

Gluconolactone is milder than gluconic acid, which is why it is especially recommended for severe pathologies such as ichthyosis. The acid (carboxyl) group in gluconolactone is "masked," and does not cause burning in contact with the skin. During hydrolysis, the ring "unfolds." The lactone turns into the α-form, gluconic acid, a substance natural to cells. By acidifying the *stratum corneum*, gluconolactone activates proteases that break down corneodesmosomes, facilitating corneocyte desquamation.

Thanks to their dermatological mildness, the PHAs can be used to care for skin with a weak barrier (atopic dermatitis, ichthyosis) and increased sensitivity. The PHAs help such skin to get rid of horny masses in time, normalize the process of cellular renewal of the epidermis, and strengthen the barrier function.

PHAs are useful for photodamaged skin, as its barrier properties have been compromised by high doses of UV radiation. Delicately acting at the level of the *stratum corneum*, PHAs help smooth out the microrelief, restore hydration, and even the skin tone.

Chapter 3
Enzymatic peels

Enzymes are specific and rather complex protein molecules that function as biological catalysts in the body. Enzymes are ubiquitous in the body, both in cells and the extracellular space. They facilitate biochemical reactions between certain substances (**substrates**) that could not react without a catalyst, or the reaction would be too slow. The substances resulting from this reaction are called **products**.

Each enzyme controls only one biochemical reaction due to its high substrate specificity, which is ensured by the enzyme's **active center** — the reaction occurs only after the substrate is bound to it. The active center of many enzymes contains a so-called **coenzyme**, a small molecule of a non-protein nature (vitamins often function as coenzymes) or metal cations (**Fig. II-3-1**).

There are thousands of biochemical reactions in a living organism, and thousands of different enzymes have been found. Although each reaction proceeds independently, they are combined into a single **metabolism**. In this complex system, the reactions involved in the syn-

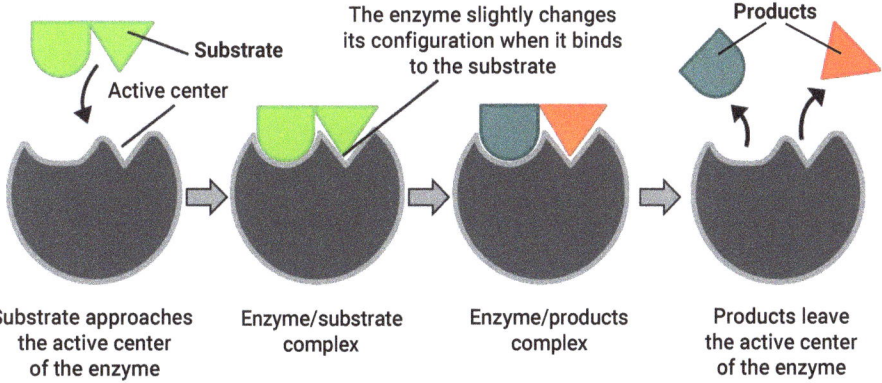

Figure II-3-1. How an enzyme works (example of a decomposition reaction)

thesis of new substances (anabolism) are balanced with those leading to the decay of old substances (catabolism). If the balance is broken, the problems begin (Ishida-Yamamoto A. et al., 2011).

The most important condition for the successful operation of an enzyme is its spatial configuration (3D structure) — if it is changed, the enzyme loses the ability to selectively bind substrate molecules, due to which the chemical reaction would not occur.

Enzyme disruption can be caused by a variety of factors. Some of the main ones are:
- Mutation of the gene encoding the enzyme
- Changes in the expression of the gene encoding the enzyme
- Chemical damage to the enzyme structure (e.g., by a keratolytic, see Part II, section 1.1)
- Coenzyme deficiency
- Substrate deficiency
- Changes in external conditions (pH, ionic strength of the aqueous medium, temperature)

Despite the absence of living cells, the *stratum corneum* shows high enzymatic activity, and many different biochemical reactions take place in it, providing barrier function. The coordinated work of the entire enzymatic ensemble is necessary to maintain the physical integrity of the *stratum corneum* while ensuring its continuous renewal (Has C., 2018). We touched on this topic in the chapter on acid peels when we discussed the pH gradient through the *stratum corneum* (see Part II, section 2.2).

In this chapter, we take a closer look at skin enzymes responsible for desquamation of corneocytes, which have become the prototype for a special category of chemical peels with proteolytic enzymes (proteases) as the active component. We will also analyze the peculiarities of formulations and applications of topical formulations containing enzymes.

3.1. *Stratum corneum*'s proteases: types and functions

Timely exfoliation of corneocytes is a prerequisite for the normal functioning of the *stratum corneum*. It begins approximately in

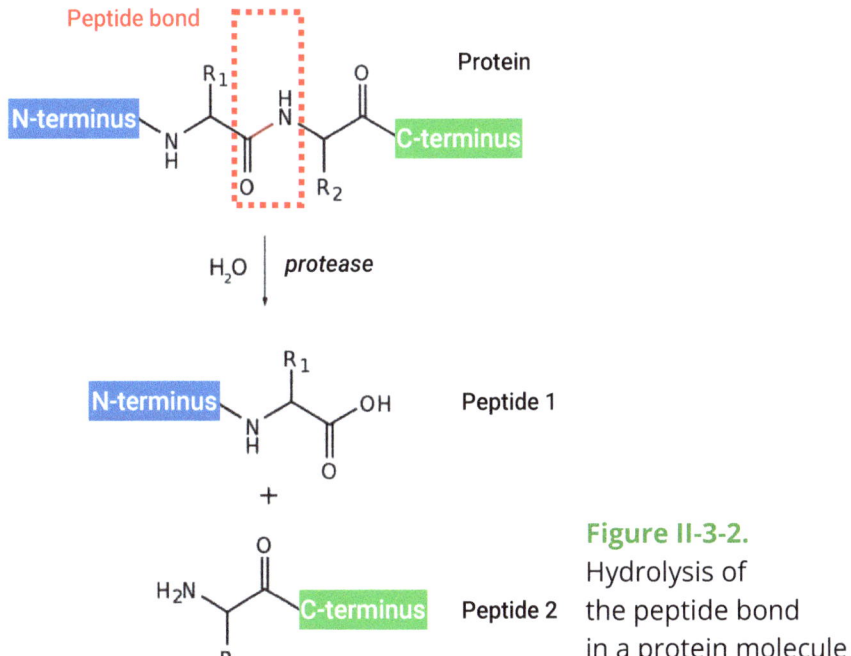

Figure II-3-2. Hydrolysis of the peptide bond in a protein molecule

the middle of the *stratum corneum* with the gradual destruction of the corneodesmosomes, which, for the time being, hold the corneocytes together. At the very top, corneodesmosomes are already destroyed, and corneocytes freely leave the skin, giving way to new ones.

A complete change in the *stratum corneum* occurs on average in 3–4 days and is driven by proteolytic enzymes (proteases), which are enzymes from the class of hydrolases that break down the peptide bonds between amino acids in proteins (**Fig. II-3-2**).

3.1.1. Proteases and antiproteases

Proteases are divided into groups according to the structure of the active center. The amino acid that forms the enzyme's active center determines the group name. Representatives of three groups of proteolytic enzymes — serine, cysteine, and aspartate — are found in the *stratum corneum*. Studies have shown that their joint work is clearly coordinated and regulated primarily by the pH gradient through the *stratum corneum* and by protease inhibitors — antiproteases.

Serine proteases

Serine proteases (representatives: kallikreins, matriptase, prostasin) are found at all levels of the *stratum corneum*, but are present in the highest quantities at the border of the *stratum corneum* and the granular layer of the epidermis.

Optimal activity of serine proteases is at neutral–alkaline pH values. If the pH tends to be 7 at the border of horny and granular layers, the pH is acidic in the upper layers. This means that **serine proteases are normally much more active at the bottom and middle of the *stratum corneum* than at its surface**. If an alkaline preparation is applied to the skin, the activity of the upper serine proteases to break down the corneodesmosomes increases, and active desquamation begins.

Serine proteases control the formation of the lipid barrier of the *stratum corneum*. Specifically, they inhibit the maturation of lamellar bodies in granular keratinocytes and inhibit acidic sphingomyelinase and β-glucocerebrosidase responsible for lipid processing (maturation) in the *stratum corneum*. Due to their inhibitory activity, the process of barrier maturation takes place at the desired speed.

Serine proteases contribute to the corneodesmosome destruction, especially in the first stages, which begin in the middle of the *stratum corneum*. Two proteases, kallikrein-5 (syn.: *stratum corneum* trypsin-like enzyme, KLK5/ SCTE) and kallikrein-7 KLK7 (syn.: *stratum corneum* chymotrypsin-like enzyme, KLK7/SCCE), have a special role here. Both enzymes are maximally expressed in the granular layer of the epidermis, then transported from the lamellar bodies into the *stratum corneum*'s intercellular space, forming a proteolytic cascade. After activation, both enzymes degrade the components of the corneodesmosomes — desmoglein, desmocollin, and corneodesmosin proteins (Caubet C. et al., 2004).

Research shows that residents of highly polluted metropolitan areas have reduced kallikrein-5 and -7 activity, which leads to the thickening of the *stratum corneum* and contributes to hyperkeratosis (Huang N. et al., 2020).

Conversely, when the activity of these proteases is pathologically high, the skin peels intensively. This, for example, is observed in Netherton syndrome (Descargues P. et al., 2006), manifesting as very dry skin and filmy scaling, along with other clinical signs. Netherton syndrome is a hereditary disease caused by a mutation in the *LEKTI* gene encoding the serine protease inhibitor type Kazal-5 (Lee A.-Y., 2020).

An increase in serine protease activity has also been proven in eczematous atopic dermatitis. In the non-eczematous form of this disease, characterized by very dry skin, the activity of serine proteases is reduced (Voegeli R. et al., 2011; Fortugno P. et al., 2012; Rawlings A.V., Voegeli R., 2013).

Abnormal activity of serine proteases of different types is observed in psoriasis patients, especially in the affected areas (Komatsu N. et al., 2007).

Another side of serine protease action is the activation of interleukin-1 precursor (pro-IL-1), stored in large quantities in the *stratum corneum*, and triggering the associated cascade of inflammatory reactions (Nylander-Lundqvist E., Egelrud T., 1997). In some cases, serine proteases can also activate the PAR-2 receptor (protease-activated receptor-2), which is a transmembrane signaling receptor for epidermal inflammation development (Pawar N.R. et al., 2019).

Aspartate proteases

The most important representative of this group of proteinases in the *stratum corneum* is cathepsin D. This enzyme is active at several sites at once. On the one hand, it participates in the formation of corneocytes by activating transglutaminase 1, the enzyme responsible for the formation of crosslinks in cornified envelope proteins — involucrin and loricrin (Egberts F. et al., 2004). On the other hand, it is involved in corneodesmosome degradation (Horikoshi T. et al., 1999; Igarashi S. et al., 2004).

Cysteine proteases

Cysteine is present in the active center of cysteine proteases, and their catalytic activity depends on its thiol (sulfhydryl) group –SH–, so these enzymes are sometimes called thiol proteases. Representatives of cysteine proteases such as cathepsins B, C, H, L, calpains, and caspases take an active part in corneal layer formation at different stages (Brocklehurst K., Philpott M.P., 2013). For example, these enzymes activate serine proteases. Therefore, it is not surprising that when their gene expression is disrupted, epidermal hyperplasia and hyperkeratosis develop in humans. Optimal conditions for the work of cysteine proteases of the *stratum corneum* are created at slightly acidic pH values of 5.0–5.5, so their participation in the destruction of corneodesmosomes is particularly noticeable near the surface of the *stratum corneum*.

Cysteine proteases are also active in the living layers of the skin, where they provide lysosomal and extracellular proteolysis of proteins (such as laminin, fibronectin, collagen, elastin), antigen presentation, prohormone processing, and remodeling of the extracellular matrix.

An interesting and practically valuable fact is that animal and plant cysteine proteases have similar characteristics, activity optimum, and substrate specificity to the *stratum corneum* proteins. This fact became the key in the search for enzymes working similarly to the skin's own proteins that would thus be suitable for topical application.

Antiproteases

Each protease has its own antiprotease. A wide variety of protease inhibitors exist both in the epidermal living layers and the *stratum corneum*'s intercellular spaces. It is antiproteases that provide fine regulation of proteolysis during desquamation. Disturbance of the protease–antiprotease balance can have dramatic consequences for the homeostasis of the whole skin (Meyer-Hoffert U., 2009). To date, a number of clinical syndromes associated with malfunctioning antiproteases in the skin have been described, such as Netherton syndrome and Papillon–Lefevre syndrome (Zeeuwen P.L., 2004; van den Bogaard E.H.J. et al., 2019).

Since cosmetic proteases are similar to the skin's proteolytic enzymes, epidermal antiproteases can also interact with peel enzymes, inhibiting or altering their activity. For example, papain work is inhibited by dermal stefins A, B, and D. Antiproteases called α2-macroglobulins interact interestingly with papain (as well as with other protease families). It was shown that when papain is systemically (orally) introduced into the body, it forms complexes with these proteins. At the same time, it does not lose but changes its properties, becomes active against low-molecular-weight substrates, becomes insensitive to other protein inhibitors, and is not subject to autolysis (Howell J.B. et al., 1983). In addition, the antigenic determinants of the papain protein molecule are masked. Consequently, they are not recognized by the components of the immune system and therefore do not exhibit antigenic properties, extending their circulation period in the body. α2-Macroglobulins are also present in the epidermis (Galliano M.F. et al., 2006), so it is possible that similar processes take place with "cosmetic" papain, and this is what ensures good tolerance of papain and its effective proteolytic effect on the skin surface.

3.1.2. Aesthetic treatments affecting the *stratum corneum*'s protease activity

If the activity of the *stratum corneum* proteases changes in one direction or another, problems arise. For example, protease activity increases in the skin of patients with atopic eczematous dermatitis and psoriasis during inflammation (including after UV irradiation). In such skin, the *stratum corneum* is thin and fragile (Cork M.J. et al., 2009; Voegeli R. et al., 2009; Elias P.M., Wakefield J.S., 2014).

In contrast, in the skin with hyperkeratosis, protease activity is reduced. Because of this, corneocytes cannot leave the skin in time, and the *stratum corneum* thickens. In particular, this occurs in some forms of ichthyosis, seborrhea, and xerosis without signs of eczema.

The activity of *stratum corneum* proteases also decreases with age (Choi E.H. et al., 2007). This effect is explained not only by the decrease in anabolic processes' efficiency but also by the decrease in the hydration level of the *stratum corneum* (proteases, as well as other enzymes, work only in an aqueous medium). As a result, conglomerates consisting of horny masses, sebum, and impurities accumulate on the skin surface, and the skin becomes dull and grayish in color.

In skincare practice, there are tools and methods that modulate the proteolytic enzyme activity. For example, the pH level in the *stratum corneum* can be changed by applying preparations with a pH different from the normal surface pH of 5.5. Such means include topical preparations with AHA — cleansers, peels, and leave-on preparations

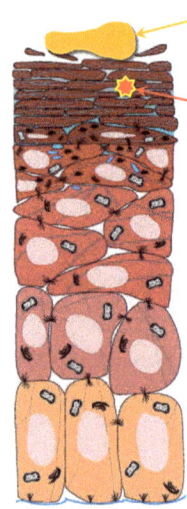

Enzymatic cleanser: removal of protein, lipid and other types of contaminants from the skin surface

Enzymatic peel: disruption of corneodesmosomes to activate desquamation

Enzymes DO NOT pass through the *stratum corneum* and work on the skin surface

Figure II-3-3. Targets for enzymatic peels and cleansers

(see Part II, chapter 2) (**Fig. II-3-3**). Selective inhibition of kallikrein-5 activity has been shown for a number of triterpenoids (e.g., ursulic and tumulose acids) from plant sources (Matsubara Y. et al., 2017).

Some physical methods can also affect the proteolytic activity of enzymes, e.g., cold plasma shower. In this case, ionized gas is the active factor — when in contact with the skin, it provokes oxidative stress in the *stratum corneum*, against which proteases are activated (Iuchi K. et al., 2018).

But there is another way, and it works when the proteolytic activity of the *stratum corneum* is reduced for one reason or another. This method consists in introducing **an extra batch of proteolytic enzymes** into the *stratum corneum* with topical agents, **which act similarly to its own proteases**. These enzymes are too large to pass through the *stratum corneum*. They do not need to because their targets, the corneodesmosomes, which they have to cut through, are located at the very surface of the *stratum corneum*. The externally introduced enzymes start working side by side with the skin's own enzymes, facilitating corneocyte desquamation to make room for new ones and ensure uninterrupted renewal of the *stratum corneum*.

If there are substances of a protein nature on the skin surface, for example, from cosmetic products, proteolytic enzymes also destroy them. That is why enzymes are included not only in peels to facilitate desquamation but also in cleansers to remove surface impurities. Enzymatic cleansers are a special category of cosmetic products and may contain enzymes that break down other organic substances (hydrocarbons and fats) along with proteolytic enzymes, but these enzymes are not suitable as peeling agents.

What are the peculiarities of enzymatic peeling? Let's find out.

3.2. Prescription features of enzymatic peels

Enzymatic peels specifically target the corneodesmosomes in the surface layers of the *stratum corneum*. Corneodesmosomes are proteins, so peeling enzymes must have primarily proteolytic activity.

3.2.1. Proteases — the main active components of enzymatic peels

Modern enzymatic peels use proteases from various sources, the most diverse being the group of plant enzymes.

Plant proteases

Plant proteases belong to the **cysteine peptidase** family (Reddy V.B., Lerner E.A., 2010).

Papain, a hydrolytic enzyme contained in all parts of the melon tree (papaya) *Carica papaya* (except the roots), is very popular; it is found in greatest amounts in immature fruits (Ajlia S.A. et al., 2010). Papain is interesting because it is the only cysteine protease with exopeptidase activity, i.e., it "bites off" the protein from the ends of the chain and can therefore break it down to its original amino acids. All other plant cysteine proteases used in skincare practice are endopeptidases, and the products of their activity are peptides of different sizes, not free amino acids. Molecular weight of papain is 20.7 kDa, i.e., it is a relatively small protein, just like most other cysteine proteases. But even such "modest" size considerably limits its penetration into the skin. Interestingly, papain needs activators to make it work. In the skin, such activators are cysteine and glutathione; in cosmetics, they can be sodium thiosulfate, thioglycolic acid, and metal chelators (for example, ethylenediaminetetraacetic acid — EDTA).

Papain can hydrolyze almost all peptide bonds, except those formed by proline residues. But it pays special "attention" to bonds formed by glycine, hydrophobic amino acids leucine and isoleucine, aromatic amino acids tyrosine and phenylalanine, as well as aspartic, glutamic, and cysteic acids. These amino acids are rich in human keratin proteins that form the *stratum corneum*, hair fibers, and nail plates (Brocklehurst K., Philpott M.P., 2013).

Besides papain, papaya's latex (milky juice) contains other cysteine proteases: chymopapains A and B, peptidases A and B, and **caricain**. These enzymes somewhat differ in physicochemical characteristics and specificity of action, but their properties are generally quite similar.

Bromelain, a mixture of cysteine proteases found in plants of the *Bromeliaceae* family, is also used in cosmetic compositions. The most studied is bromelain from pineapple stems. In this plant, the enzymes **ananain** and **comosain** were also found (Maurer H.R., 2001).

In modern enzymatic peels, **ficin** (obtained from the milky sap of the fig tree *Ficuscarica*), **actinidain** (from kiwi), **aleurain** (from barley), as well as proteases from mango, pumpkin, yam, and other plants are used.

In papaya, pineapple, and some other plants, in addition to proteases, other enzymes are present — amylases (amylolytic enzymes that hydrolyze α-(1,4)-glycoside bond in amylose, amylopectic glycogen and other maltooligosaccharides), lysozyme (a hydrolase that breaks down bacterial walls), and lipases (involved in the breakdown of fats, which are esters of glycerol and higher fatty acids). Plant lipases are mainly found in seeds, fruits, tubers, rhizomes of cereals, crucifers, and legumes. Lipases have been found in papaya and pineapple. When skin peels based on the so-called plant "pulp" are applied to the skin, the lipase contained in it works synergistically with proteases, destroying intercellular lipids of the *stratum corneum* and allowing proteases to penetrate deeper into it. Lysozyme also provides antibacterial skin protection.

Proteases of microbial origin

Microbial proteases **belong to the class of serine proteases**; their active center contains the amino acid serine. It should be noted that the activity and diversity of bacterial proteases are much higher than that of plant proteases. This is because proteases are the main survival tool for microbes, a means of invasion into the host tissues and spreading throughout its body. In addition, there are as many hosts as there are specific conditions to which they need to adapt. Therefore, one such enzyme, **subtilisin (subtilopeptidase)**, a product of *Bacillus subtilis* metabolism, acts less specifically than papain, breaking down more diverse proteins, and is consequently more effective at removing protein contaminants. The FDA has deemed isolated and purified subtilisin safe for use in food, detergents, and cosmetics.

Different strains of *Bacillus subtilis* and some other microorganisms are used to produce subtilisin, and the extraction, purification, and stabilization of the enzyme also vary among manufacturers (Karlsson C. et al., 2007). Therefore, the output enzyme products are not identical in properties. Each manufacturer gives its product a unique brand name to distinguish it from its counterparts. Still, it is not yet a ready-to-use substance, but only a single component that is later incorporated into the final cosmetic product.

For example, an enzyme product called travase (Travase®) is included in topical medicinal formulations for rapidly clearing scabs from wounds — such preparations are used in anti-burn therapy.

Keratoline (Keratoline®) is another subtilisin-based product adapted for use in cosmetics. It has subtilisin dissolved in a liquid aqueous gel with a small amount of glycerin and propylene glycol to stabilize the enzyme and to facilitate its introduction into the complex composition.

Proteases of animal origin

Animal proteases can be found in cosmetic peels: aspartate proteases — **pepsin** and serine proteases — **trypsin**, **chymotrypsin**, and **pancreatin**. However, the general trend away from using ingredients of animal origin in favor of biotechnological and plant components, as well as the lower stability of animal proteases, has resulted in their increasing absence from cosmetic formulations.

The well-known collagenase is successfully used in medicine for debridement — cleaning wounds from tissue decay products. Treating wounds with proteolytic enzymes accelerates their healing, preventing infection and forming rough scars. It should be remembered that, in the case of wounds, the drug is applied to the skin deprived of its barrier, which means that there is no problem of enzyme penetration through the *stratum corneum*. We are unaware of any approved peel/exfoliation product containing this enzyme.

Modified natural peptidases

Modified enzymes are more stable than the natural ones. For example, crosslinked papain (cross-papain) was developed by specialists at BASF. The individual molecules of the enzyme are cross-linked with a heat-stable crosslinking agent so that their active centers remain available for reaction with the substrate. Such an aggregate of several enzyme units is attached to a polymer substrate. The result is a complex with high enzymatic activity. The complexes are immersed in sodium alginate gel for additional stabilization (**Fig. II-3-4**).

Cross-papain withstands high temperatures, and its individual enzyme units become resistant even to surfactants, making its inclusion into emulsions possible. This is a great advantage because naturally unmodified proteases can only be incorporated into aqueous solutions or gels that do not contain surface-active emulsifiers.

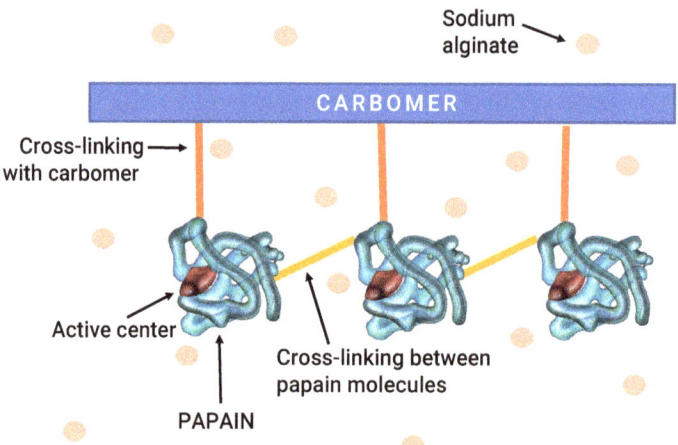

Figure II-3-4. Example of a modified enzyme, cross-papain

3.2.2. How to keep the enzyme active

Enzymes are very capricious substances and, due to their chemical nature, rapidly inactivate when external conditions deviate from the optimum. All enzymes are characterized by peptide chains that are packed in space in a certain way. Both the primary amino acid sequence of the protein chain and its spatial structure, stabilized by strong chemical (mostly disulfide) and weak hydrogen bonds, are important. There are also hydrophobic interactions (**Fig. II-3-5**).

- Ionic bonds are easily broken by heat, changes in solution pH, and ionic composition.
- The chemical bonds are broken down in the presence of surfactants, keratolytics, and other proteolytic enzymes.
- Hydrophobic interactions — their nature varies depending on the external environment (they are strongest in solution, adding hydrophobic substances weakens them).

Therefore, heating should not be used in the production of enzyme preparations. Care is also needed when choosing other substances to include in the finished formulation.

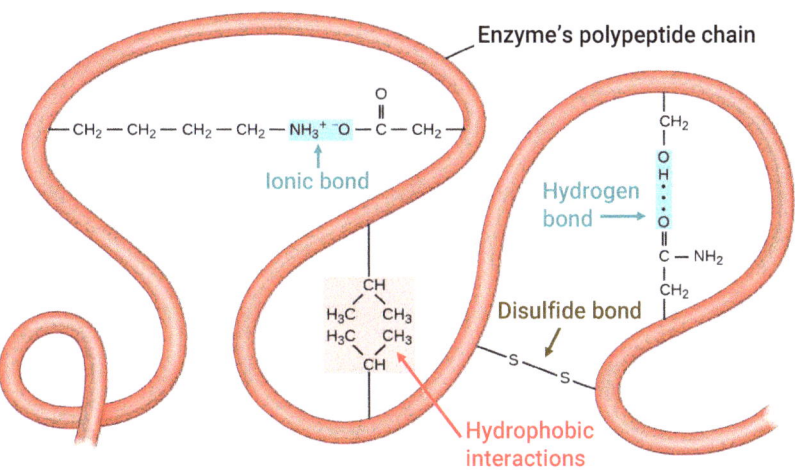

Figure II-3-5. Intramolecular bonds stabilize the spatial configuration of a protein

The aim is not only to preserve the enzyme structure, but also to protect it from microorganisms because it is an organic protein molecule, which is a delicacy for most microbes. Therefore, all enzyme preparations must contain **preservatives**.

To ensure that the enzyme is active in the finished formulation, the following rules must be followed during production:
- Do not heat the enzyme
- Avoid combinations with emulsifiers or alcohol
- Maintain a pH of 5–6
- Use with caution substances that dissociate in water (salts)
- Use preservatives to protect the finished product from microbial breakdown

3.2.3. Combining enzymes with other peeling agents in one formulation

Formulations in which proteolytic enzymes are combined with other peeling agents can be found on the market. Each such combination has to be considered individually and in light of the following questions:
1. How realistic is it technologically — will the active substances retain their activity in the finished product?
2. How justified is it biologically — will these substances work in synergy?

Enzymes + salicylic acid
Let's look at the combination of proteolytic enzymes and salicylic acid. Salicylic acid is oil-soluble, and enzymes are water-soluble. An aqueous gel or solution form is not suitable because salicylic acid will precipitate. An anhydrous ointment base is not suitable either because there is no room for water-soluble enzymes.

An emulsion variant (cream) with both aqueous and oil phases could be suitable if it were not for emulsifiers, without which an emulsion cannot exist. Unfortunately, in addition to stabilizing the emulsion, most emulsifiers affect the 3D configuration of protein molecules, leading to enzyme inactivation. So, it all comes down to finding a suitable emulsifier in the case of an emulsion base. This leaves the powder option, a dry mixture of substances diluted with a special aqueous solution just before application. The salicylic acid will not have time to precipitate, and the enzyme will be in an appropriate aqueous environment and will be active.

In addition to the difficulty of combining water- and oil-soluble substances, there is one more factor to consider: salicylic acid, being keratolytic, can disrupt the enzyme structure by breaking disulfide bonds (see Part II, section 1.1). Therefore, the possibility of combining salicylic acid with a natural enzyme is highly questionable. But with a modified enzyme of the cross-papain type, it is justified because such an enzyme complex is much more resistant to the keratolytic action.

In terms of biological relevance, both salicylic acid and proteases target corneodesmosomes. Salicylic acid breaks disulfide bonds and unfolds the protein chain of the corneodesmosomes, making it more accessible to fragmentation by proteases. Combining salicylic acid with proteases reduces the concentration of both salicylic acid and enzymes in the formulation without compromising the overall keratolytic effectiveness of the drug (**Fig. II-3-6**).

Combined keratolytic peel **is especially recommended for very dry seborrheic skin with hyperkeratosis**, of course, if it is possible to solve technical issues during its creation.

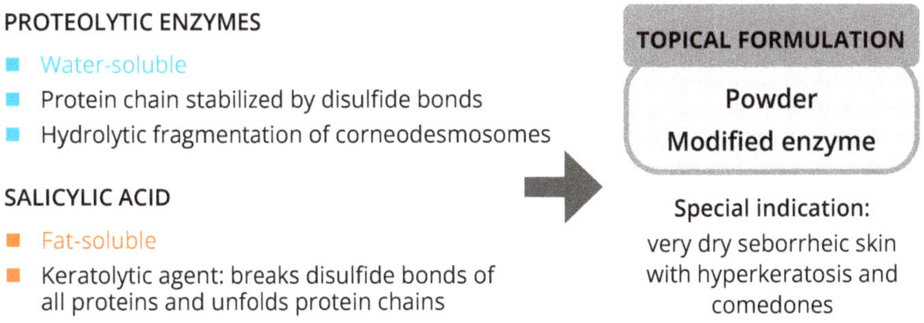

PROTEOLYTIC ENZYMES
- Water-soluble
- Protein chain stabilized by disulfide bonds
- Hydrolytic fragmentation of corneodesmosomes

SALICYLIC ACID
- Fat-soluble
- Keratolytic agent: breaks disulfide bonds of all proteins and unfolds protein chains

TOPICAL FORMULATION
Powder
Modified enzyme

Special indication:
very dry seborrheic skin with hyperkeratosis and comedones

Figure II-3-6. Combination of proteolytic enzymes and salicylic acid in one formulation

Enzymes + AHAs

Combining proteolytic enzymes with AHAs is easier because AHAs are also water-soluble. Such a combined preparation can be in the form of an aqueous solution or gel. As emulsifiers are not needed here, we can take natural, unmodified enzymes.

But there is another problem. The peeling power of the AHAs is related to the pH of the solution — the lower it is, the more effective the peel is. In acid peels, the pH is lower than 3. The **proteolytic enzymes used for peels, on the contrary, are active at pH 5–6**. A dilemma arises — if we want to use an acid peel with a pH < 3, the simultaneous inclusion of enzymes becomes meaningless because they will be inactivated.

Still, there are products on the market that combine enzymes with AHAs. Their pH is around 5 to allow the enzymes to work. Lactic and citric acids are the most common AHA forms in these preparations due to their specific action (see Part II, section 2.3). Lactic acid is a good moisturizer and is part of the natural moisturizing factor, so its addition to enzymatic peels is especially indicated for dry aging skin, characterized by NMF decrease. Citric acid lightens pigmentation, so preparations containing it are especially recommended for skin with pigmented spots (**Fig. II-3-7**).

Such combination formulations **are recommended for sebaceous dry skin with fine wrinkles and uneven tone**.

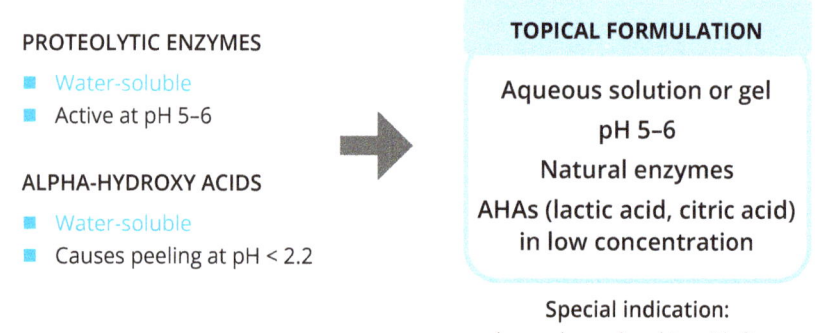

Figure II-3-7. Combination of proteolytic enzymes and AHAs in one formulation

The presence of enzymes in the formulation is not a guarantee that the finished product will exhibit enzymatic activity. For an enzymatic peel to work, the manufacturer needs to consider many nuances, such as:
1. Proteolytic enzymes are the main active ingredient; other enzymes can play an auxiliary role, but can be omitted.
2. A suitable base for the drug is an aqueous solution/gel or powder that is diluted with a special solution before use and not stored.
3. The pH of the base or solution used to dilute the powder should be in the 5–6 range.
4. Careful combination with other active ingredients and peeling agents, which must be evaluated from a technical and biological point of view.
5. Obligatory presence of a preservative (in the case of a prepared solution or gel, which is stored).
6. Avoid heating at all stages of work with the enzyme.

3.3. Clinical effects

Although superficial enzymatic peeling does not remove deep wrinkles, scars, and age spots, it is absolutely realistic to revitalize the skin and improve its condition and appearance. Immediately after the enzymatic peeling, the skin looks fresher and brighter. This visual effect is due to the rapid and delicate removal of the most superficial corneocytes, which make the skin rough.

Electron microscopy can be used to show how the skin surface differs after enzymatic and acid peel treatments.

Scales can be seen on the skin before the treatment. Their edges are already raised and move away from the skin, but not completely. After enzymatic peeling, the surface looks polished — such a smooth surface reflects light differently than a rough surface, so the skin immediately becomes bright and shiny after enzymatic peeling. There is no visible scaling — neither during the procedure (as in the case of keratolytic peels) nor after several days, as in the case of acid and retinol

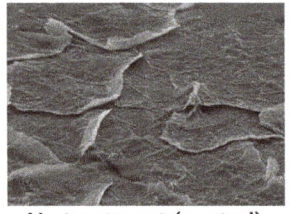 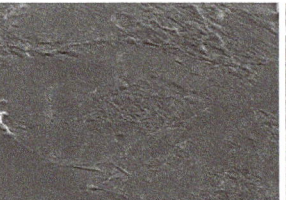 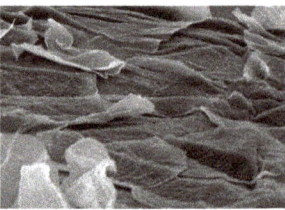

No treatment (control)   Treated with Keratoline™   Treated with AHAs

Figure II-3-8. Electron microscopy of the skin surface (Keratoline™ / Sederma)

peeling (**Fig. II-3-8**). For comparison, consider the skin after the treatment with acid peels. Its scales are initially floppy and do not immediately leave the surface. Skin scaling after acid peeling starts after a few days, which is due to the specific mechanism of their action.

Clean, fresh skin is the first aspect that catches the eye after the procedure, which the beautician's clients like very much. But there are also "deeper" effects of the enzymes contained in the peel formulations. Intense exfoliation that occurs under the action of peels, although slight, is still an injury to the skin. As previously discussed, any injury signals the activation of reparative processes, replacing the old cells with new ones. Therefore, although enzymatic peels work on the surface, their "echoes" inevitably occur in all skin layers.

One of the mechanisms determining such a "remote" effect is a special signaling system existing within the *stratum corneum* and in the upper layers of the epidermis: calcium ion concentration gradient (Lee A.-Y., 2020).

This signaling system stimulates the keratinocytes' lipid-synthesizing activity of the granular layer in response to skin damage. It works approximately as follows: when the barrier is breached under the influence of enzymatic peels and water ingress into the skin, calcium concentration in the surrounding granular keratinocytes declines sharply, and this is a signal for activation of lamellar cell secretion. The result is a rapid restructuring of the epidermal metabolism and the skin lipid barrier restoration.

An important additional benefit of enzymatic peels is the slowing down of facial hair growth. As women age, this problem becomes increasingly disturbing. Proteases, penetrating the open mouths of hair follicles, destroy the hair keratin and slow down its growth, thinning the hair shaft. This effect becomes especially noticeable after a course of peels.

The use of enzymatic peel increases the effectiveness of cosmetic products applied after the procedure: by loosening the uppermost and toughest layer of dead cells, proteases facilitate deeper penetration of other active ingredients.

3.4. Practical aspects

3.4.1. Indications and contraindications

In general, the indications for enzymatic peeling, as well as for chemical peels of other categories, are epidermal problems related to impaired keratinization or pigmentation (see Part I, section 1.1). Enzymatic peeling is especially effective in cases with leading signs of keratinization disorders, which form **a syndrome of dry skin** — roughness, keratosis areas, visible scaling, superficial wrinkles.

It is important to recognize that signs of dryness can occur in skin with any level of sebaceous gland activity — both low-sebum and oily (seborrheic), and in the skin with normal sebum levels. **In the case of enzymatic peeling, the oiliness of the skin does not matter — these peels can be used with any level of sebum activity**; this is an important distinction from keratolytic peels (these are salicylic and Jessner peels), for which sebum is a contraindication (see Part II, chapter 2).

Hyperkeratosis occurs when the skin's enzymes cannot provide timely exfoliation. This occurs in (**Fig. II-3-9**):
- People over 50 years of age against the background of changes in hormonal regulation
- Photoaging
- Seborrhea, hyperkeratosis of the estuaries of the hair follicles is one of the stages in the pathogenesis of acne
- Dry low-sebum skin due to a water deficit in the *stratum corneum* — this condition can occur in non-eczematous atopic dermatitis and psoriasis, in the case of improper selection of cleansers and cosmetic care products, in prolonged stress
- Ichthyosis

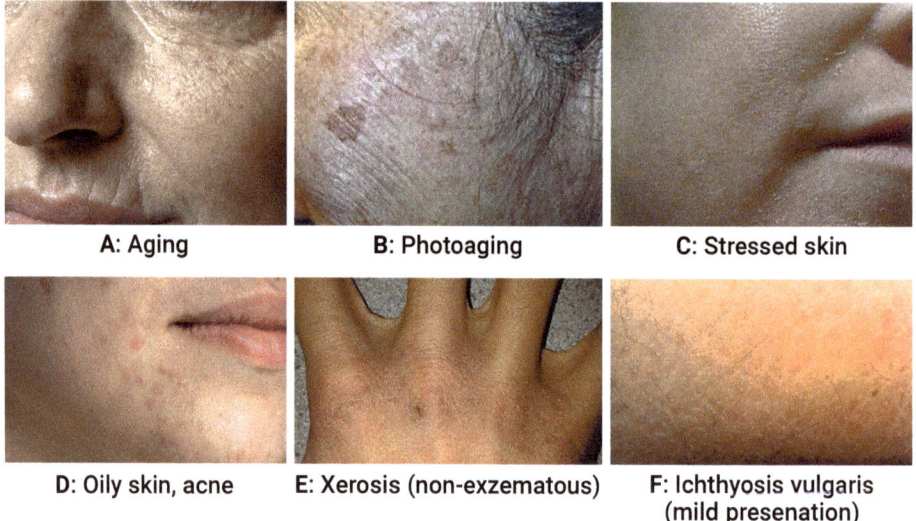

Figure II-3-9. Indications for enzymatic peeling
(Images by: A–D — Freepik.com, E, F — Wikipedia.com)

With all these different conditions and diseases, **there is a decrease in proteolytic activity in the *stratum corneum*, so reinforcement in the form of external enzymes would be justified**.

On the contrary, **enzymatic peeling is contraindicated in cases of increased proteolytic activity of the *stratum corneum***. Such cases include (**Fig. II-3-10**):

- Atopic dermatitis and psoriasis — skin diseases in which the *stratum corneum* is thin and misshapen, including due to the high activity of proteolytic enzymes
- Diabetes mellitus — a hormonal disease that increases the activity of proteolytic enzymes
- Foci of chronic inflammation, as the structure of the *stratum corneum* above them is thin
- Inflammatory dermatoses, including infectious and autoimmune
- In open wound, a cut, or an abrasion, as the *stratum corneum* must first regenerate

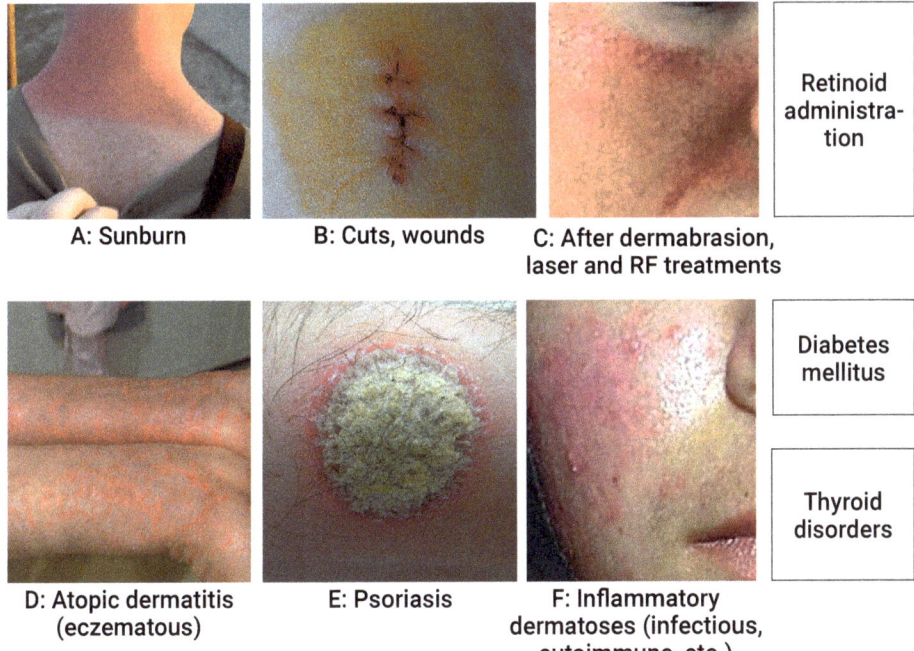

Figure II-3-10. Contraindications for enzymatic peeling (Image by Wikipedia.com)

- After UV exposure
- After a photoprocedure, even a non-ablative (e.g., IPL rejuvenation)
- After aesthetic procedures that damage the *stratum corneum* (e.g., dermabrasion, microneedling, fractional laser or radiofrequency/RF-thermolysis)

Intolerance to any of the peel components is also a contraindication. After all, enzymes are proteins, and proteins are known to be the most common cause of allergies. Therefore, an allergy test should be performed when the enzymatic preparation is used for the first time.

Vigilance is also necessary when using retinoids, as these substances accelerate the cellular renewal of the epidermis and thin the *stratum corneum*. Thus, if we also accelerate desquamation with enzymes, the barrier properties of the *stratum corneum* can weaken considerably, which leads to increased skin sensitivity and irritability.

3.4.2. How to perform enzymatic peeling

The manufacturer's instructions must be followed diligently regardless of where the procedure is performed — in salons, beauty clinics, or at home.

In addition, the peculiarities of the enzymatic peeling should also be considered.

1. Allergy testing is mandatory when using any enzymatic peel for the first time.
2. Refraining from products containing glycolic acid, salicylic acid, and retinol the day before and the day after the peel is mandatory.
3. The peel product is applied to cleaned and well-moisturized skin because **the enzymes need water to work**! For this purpose, you can use warm water or, after cleansing, rub the skin with a tonic with pH 5.5–6.0.
4. Enzymatic peels can be used on any area of the body, but the zone at least 0.5 cm from the border of the eyes or other mucous membranes must be avoided. Peel formulations are never applied to open wounds, to skin shaved less than 24 hours before the procedure, or to skin after dermabrasion (see the contraindications above).
5. While the preparation remains on the skin, it is recommended to cover the treated areas with a warm damp towel — this is done so that the water from the preparation does not evaporate, and the skin remains sufficiently moisturized.
6. Exposure time varies from 10 minutes to half an hour for different preparations and different skin conditions — here, it is important to follow the manufacturer's recommendations.
7. To remove the preparation, it is necessary to wash the skin thoroughly with warm water. **Neutralization is not required**

even if the enzymatic peel contains AHAs because the pH of the product will not be lower than 4. If the instructions say that neutralization is mandatory, it means that the enzymes in this product are inactive, and you did not perform an enzymatic peeling but an acidic peeling.
8. Next, a moisturizer is applied to the skin, which may contain components of a natural moisturizing factor.
9. The patient should be advised not to touch the skin for one day after the procedure.
10. When going outdoors after the procedure, sunscreen should be applied.

Enzymatic peeling is a gentle procedure, after which there are no unwanted reactions in the form of persistent redness or swelling. On the contrary, the skin becomes smoother, has a beautiful shine, and looks refreshed after the procedure. Therefore, enzymatic peeling is suitable for an express procedure that does not require any recovery time.

But it can also be carried out as part of a structural skin rejuvenation program. On average, such a course includes 5–8 sessions. The frequency of treatment depends on the skin condition:
- Seborrheic skin: 2–3 times a week
- Skin with normal or slightly reduced sebum secretion, as well as for aging skin: once a week
- Very dry and sensitive skin: once every 7–10 days

If the preparation contains acids, the interval between treatments should be increased. The break between courses should be at least three months.

3.4.3. How enzymatic exfoliants are combined with AHA-based peels

The mechanisms that trigger hydroxy acid and protease activity in the epidermis and the *stratum corneum* are different, but perfectly complement and reinforce each other's effects. Therefore, if a patient's skin can withstand the effects of AHAs, a combination of acidic and enzymatic peeling is an excellent choice. Usually, these types of peels are alternated. The session frequency and the exposure duration are determined individually for each patient, depending on their skin condition.

Enzymatic peeling can also help when the patient's skin "gets used to" glycolic peels. Their effect gradually wears off, and the doctor has to use higher and higher acid concentrations. In this situation, switching to an enzymatic peel will help the skin reactions to return to the desired level.

For most (but not all!) people, enzymatic peeling is a comfortable, gentle, and safe procedure suitable for all skin phototypes.

Enzymatic peeling would be more accurately called enzymatic exfoliation because it removes only the very top corneocytes and protein impurities from the skin surface. If it is done correctly, the visible effect — glowing and lighter skin — will appear first, so it is better than other peels as an express procedure for "going out." Enzymatic peeling fits well into the general program of supporting and rejuvenating skincare at any age.

Chapter 4
Retinol peels

Retinol peels are fundamentally different from keratolytic, acidic, and enzymatic peels in that they stimulate rather than damage their targets. This is the only category of chemical peels for which the targets are living cells, more precisely, their nuclei. Retinoids are substances regulating the expression of various genes, which serve as the levers that trigger the cellular and tissue response to retinoids.

To better understand what happens in the skin when retinoids are used topically, why the skin starts to peel and renew, why sebum production decreases, and why it can become dry, let's look at the chemical nature of retinol and the biological mechanisms of its action.

4.1. Retinol and its derivatives: structure, metabolism, mechanism of action

Retinol (true vitamin A) is an oil-soluble vitamin that belongs to the organic alcohols (–OH). In the form of alcohol, it is found only in animal products. In plant-based foods, it is present in the form of β-carotene (precursor of vitamin A). In cells, it is converted to the active form — retinoic acid (RA).

4.1.1. Retinol — the first in the series of vitamins

The people of the Arctic region have had an unwritten law for centuries — never, under any circumstances, eat a polar bear's liver. They even warned the white aliens about it. But the latter, as a rule, did not listen to them, and having killed a bear, the first thing they did was to eat the liver. For this, the spirits punished them severely. Those who broke the law were afflicted with a terrible disease: they writhed with stomach cramps and vomiting, suffered from diarrhea, fell from dizziness, and went mad with a headache. After a while, their skin would begin to peel off. Witnesses said that the skin on these unfortunates' soles fell off like plaster, and they could not move until they had new skin.

And now, from the cold Arctic, let's move to the hot countries where there are no polar bears or even brown bears and where the liver is treated more respectfully. Ancient manuscripts testify that ancient Egyptians treated blindness with lotions of chicken liver juice. In ancient Greece, skin diseases were fought with liver compresses while eating the liver as food.

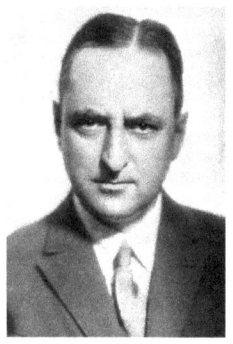

Wilhelm Stepp
(1882–1964)

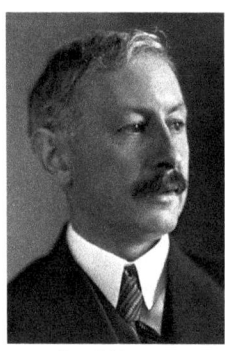

Paul Karrer
(1889–1971)

The sad experience of the Eskimos and the successful one of the Egyptians could be explained only in the twentieth century. The history of amazing discoveries began in 1909 when German scientist Wilhelm Stepp isolated a oil-soluble factor necessary for embryo development from egg yolk and then from milk. In 1920, the substance was named vitamin A.

In 1930, the Swiss organic chemist Paul Karrer determined the structure of β-carotene and proved that it is a precursor of vitamin A, for which he was subsequently awarded the Nobel Prize. In the same year, T. Moore synthesized retinol from carotenoids and began to study its effect on the body. Only in 1943 was it finally proven that it was retinol that was responsible for the misfortunes of the intrepid Arctic explorers and the last hope of the blind Egyptians. An article by Moore and Rohdal (1943), published in the Biochemical Journal, was sensational. It turned out that polar bear liver contains so much retinol (18,000–27,000 IU/g) that consumption of even a small piece (say, 250 g) exceeds the daily retinol allowance by more than 1000 times.

Retinol deficiency is just as dangerous as retinol excess. Insufficient retinol intake eventually leads to irreversible loss of vision, reduced resistance to infection, skin problems, and even death. Scientists have named the substances necessary for normal functioning and even for the very existence of the human body as vitamins (lat. *vita* — life) to emphasize their importance. **Retinol was the first among them, receiving the honorary title of vitamin A.**

4.1.2. Retinol transformations in the body and the cell

We get vitamin A from food. Animal products (e.g., liver, fish oil, egg yolk, milk, butter) contain retinol. Plants do not synthesize retinol but are a source of pro-retinol — the plant pigment β-carotene. In the intestinal mucosa cells, β-carotene is broken down into two retinol molecules with the help of the enzyme dioxygenase, which is then reduced to retinol (**Fig. II-4-1**). The amount of retinol synthesized is strictly regulated to prevent body intoxication. Retinol enters the liver

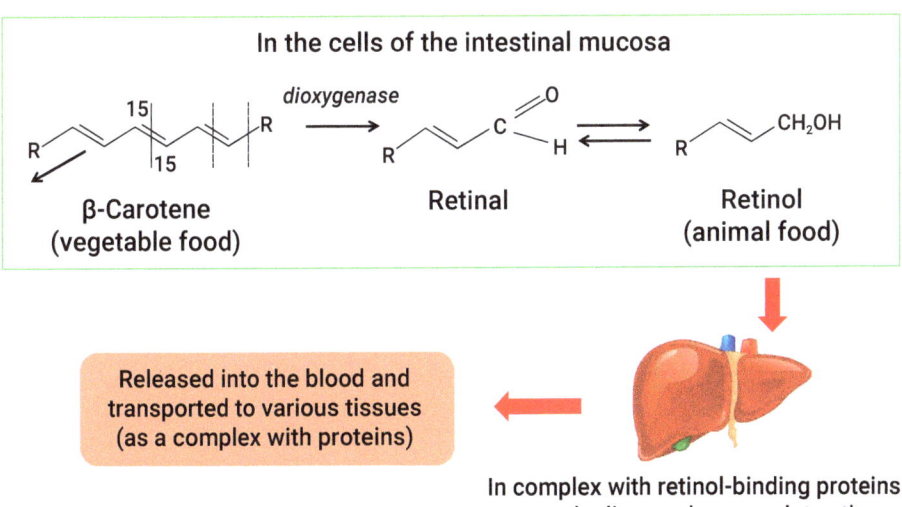

Figure II-4-1. Biotransformation of vitamin A in the body

from the intestines, where it is deposited in the stellate cells, mainly in the form of esters. The blood retinol, combined with special transport proteins, is delivered to other organs, including the skin (Zanotti G., Berni R., 2004; Blomhoff R., Blomhoff H.K., 2006; Napoli J.L., 2017).

The biologically active form is not retinol itself, but its derivative — *trans*-retinoic acid (*trans*-RA, better known among practitioners as tretinoin), formed in the cells in two steps: first, retinol is oxidized to retinal, and it, in turn, is oxidized to *trans*-RA. Another retinol derivative with physiological activity, 9-*cis*-RA, is formed from *trans*-RA (**Fig. II-4-2**). It is also possible to inactivate retinol to inactive metabolites (**Fig. II-4-3**).

The role of retinol as a chromophore in the process of visual perception was established several decades ago. This process is based on successive transformations of the retinol molecule under the influence of light.

Somewhat later, it was found that retinol affects the differentiation of epithelial cells. Today, it has already been proven that vitamin A is involved in the regulation and proliferation of many cell types from

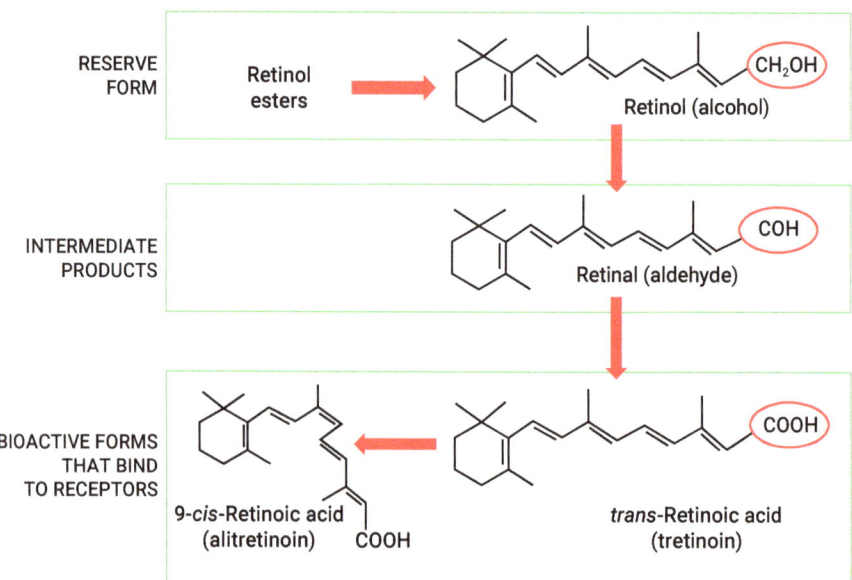

Figure II-4-2. Biotransformation of vitamin A in the cell: transformation of natural retinoids inside the cell from inactive precursors to active forms that can bind to nuclear receptors

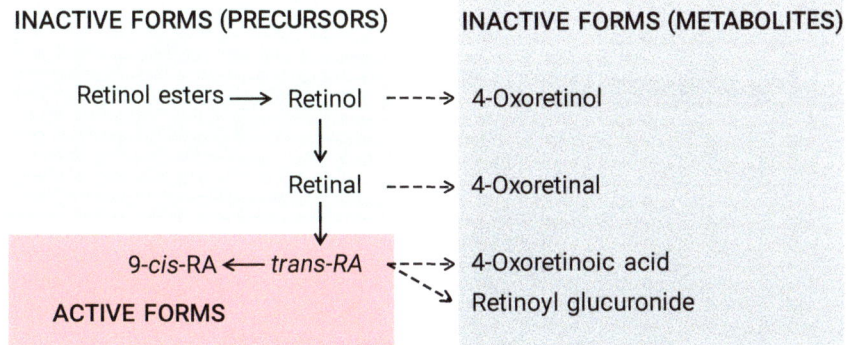

Figure II-4-3. Intracellular (endogenous) retinoids: precursors represent the stock of retinol in the cell, and metabolites result from inactivation and utilization of retinoids by the cell

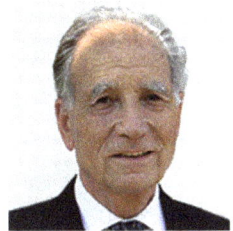

Pierre Chambon

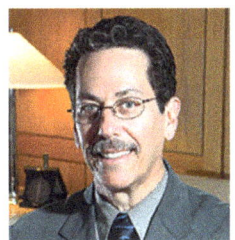

Ronald Evans

the embryonic setting and throughout life. However, this side of retinol action remained unclear until 1987, when almost simultaneously two laboratories, the French one headed by Pierre Chambon and the American one headed by Ronald Evans, discovered the receptors for *trans*-RA located in cell nuclei (Petkovich M. et al., 1987). This discovery was a turning point in the fate of vitamin A, and since then, a whole army of geneticists, molecular biologists, and biochemists have taken up the study (Evans R.M., Mangelsdorf D.J., 2014).

Cells are very sensitive to retinol concentration, and any slight deviation from the norm affects their vital functions. The mechanism of cellular regulation of retinoid metabolism is a complex and well-established system. It includes many enzymes and binding proteins that ensure retinoid capture, metabolism, deposition, and transport inside the cell.

After penetrating the plasma membrane inside the cell, retinoids are metabolized to active derivatives and bind to special proteins. In this form, they are delivered to the nucleus, where they are recognized by retinoid

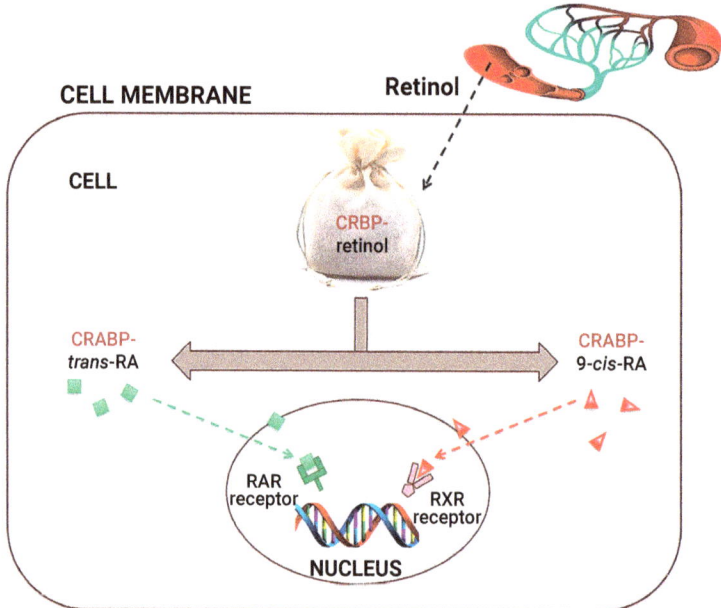

Figure II-4-4. Regulation of retinol levels in the cell

Intracellular retinoid-binding proteins:
- CRBP (cellular retinol-binding protein) — retinol deposition in the cell
- CRABP (cellular retinoic acid-binding protein) — retinoic acid delivery to the nucleus.

Each class of intracellular retinoid-binding proteins has types 1 and 2.

receptors (**Fig. II-4-4**). The activated receptor, in turn, binds to a short deoxyribonucleic acid (DNA) sequence in close proximity to the target genes' promoter and stabilizes the transcription factor (**Fig. II-4-5**). The role of the transcription factor is to ensure that the ribonucleic acid (RNA) polymerase II enzyme binds to the promoter and triggers transcription.

The above scheme is greatly simplified; in reality, everything is more complicated. Retinoic acid receptors are divided into two groups — RARs (retinoic acid receptors) and RXRs (retinoid X receptors), each having three subgroups (α, β, γ). Thus, the retinoic acid receptor system includes six types of receptors.

As for intracellular retinoid-binding proteins, there are two major classes — CRBP (cellular retinol-binding proteins) and CRABP (cellular retinoic acid-binding proteins). Each class of proteins has subclasses designated by Roman numerals I and II. These proteins are highly specific and

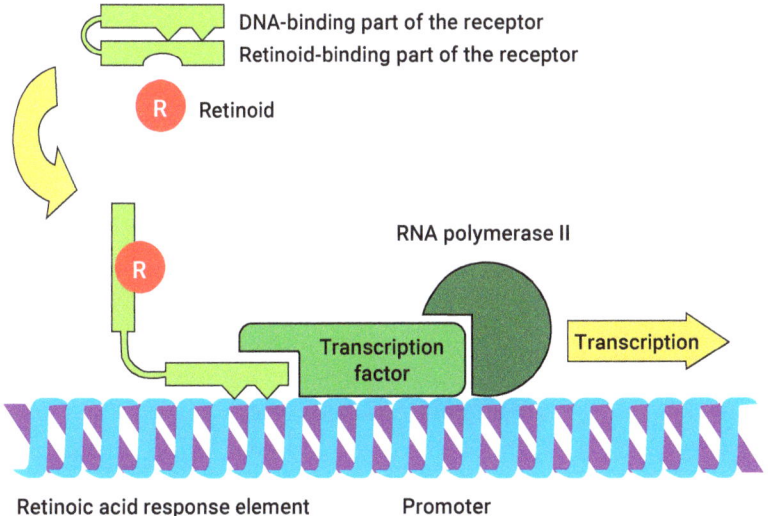

Figure II-4-5. Activation of target gene expression by retinoic receptors

Retinoid receptors:
- RARs (retinoic acid receptors)
- RXRs (retinoid X receptors)

Each receptor family has three receptor isoforms (α, β, γ)

show great affinity to their ligands (retinol and retinoic acid, respectively). The exact function of these proteins is still unclear. It is assumed that CRBPs play an important role in retinoid metabolism and deposit retinol in the cell. As for CRABPs, they presumably perform transport functions and deliver *trans*-RA to the nucleus, where it binds to its receptor.

The presence of nuclear receptors and similarities in the molecular mechanisms of activation give scientists reason to put retinol on par with the steroid and thyroid hormones since their action is also mediated through nuclear receptors. Moreover, the nuclear receptors for retinoids, steroids, and thyroids are similar in structure and mechanism of action and can even influence each other's activity. This explains, in particular, the fact that vitamin D (steroid precursor) acts synergistically with vitamin A, stimulating its uptake and metabolism in keratinocytes.

4.1.3. Synthetic retinoids

Over time, scientists have found substances that have similar effects to vitamin A. Synthetic and natural compounds with a mechanism of action similar to retinol began to be called retinoids and used to treat a variety of diseases, including skin diseases (Krężel W. et al., 2019). **Fig. II-4-6** shows examples of retinoids used in clinical practice. The first-generation retinoids are natural compounds because they are retinol derivatives found in cells. The other substances are not found in nature and are classified as synthetic retinoids.

The fourth-generation retinoids — selectinoid G and tripharotene — are considered promising for dermatology. Both are selective agonists of RAR-γ, the most common receptor type for retinoic acid in the skin. Seletinoid G appeared earlier on the market and has proven

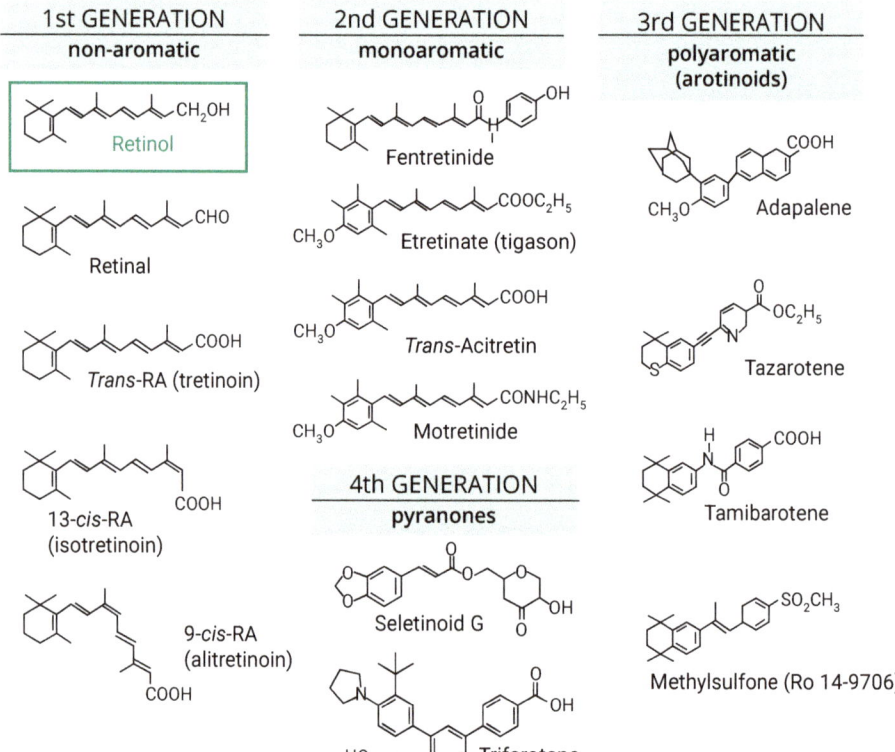

Figure II-4-6. Retinoids in clinical practice

to be quite good at improving the healing and remodeling of the dermal matrix. The patent for this retinoid belongs to the Korean company AmorePacific, and it can be found in anti-aging beauty products belonging mainly to Asian brands.

At the end of 2019, another representative of the fourth generation of retinoids received FDA approval — tripharotene (developed by Galderma), registered under the trade name Aklief. The first publications about the new retinoid appeared in 2018 in the British Journal of Dermatology (Balak D.M.W., 2018). According to this study, tripharotene has almost all the therapeutic properties of classical retinoids (anti-inflammatory, comedolytic, and depigmenting) but causes fewer unpleasant side effects, such as irritation and flaking, due to its selective binding to RAR-γ. In addition, tripharotene has an interesting metabolism: according to the manufacturer, it is stable in human keratinocytes for 24 hours but is almost immediately destroyed by hepatocytes, which limits the risks of its systemic effects. Therefore, it can be used on large areas of the skin, which is one of the main advantages of the drug. The fight against extensive acne lesions is considered the main indication for its use — the FDA has approved the use of Aclif for treating acne on the face and the body (chest, back, and shoulders). However, this retinoid is not approved for use in cosmetics, including peels.

4.1.4. Plant retinoids

Plants do not synthesize retinoids. However, they have substances that can be converted into retinol in the human body or have a retinol-like effect on cells.

The first group includes β-carotene — it is converted to retinol in the body when ingested orally, i.e., it is pro-vitamin A. This transformation occurs in the intestinal cells, as they have the necessary enzyme for this — dioxygenase. When applied topically, β-carotene in the skin remains β-carotene because skin cells do not have this enzyme. β-Carotene has no affinity to nuclear retinoid receptors, which means that it cannot influence the cell's genetic apparatus the way retinoids do. But this does not mean that β-carotene and carotenoids, in general, are useless in cosmetics. They are good antioxidants that help the skin to resist oxidative stress and increase its resistance to

UV rays (Stahl W., Sies H., 2012). When applied topically, you should not expect them to have the clinical effects typical of retinoids. If the cream container is labeled "plant provitamin A" and the list of ingredients includes carotene, it is just a marketing ploy.

The second group includes substances that can bind to nuclear retinoid receptors (Chaudhuri R.K., Bojanowski K., 2014). This binding is much weaker than that of retinoids and the clinical effects (including adverse reactions) are not as pronounced as those of real retinoids, but they will still act on cells similarly to retinoids. Bacuchiol, derived from psoralea witch hazel seeds, belongs to this group. Today, this substance is popular and can be found in products for the correction of age-related changes and for skin with increased sebum production (Dhaliwal S. et al., 2019).

4.1.5. How to explain the variety of clinical effects of retinoids

The intracellular lever that retinoids act on is a gene (or several genes, given that there are several types of receptors) that starts to be expressed when retinoid receptors are activated. The clinical manifestations of retinoids are so diverse that it is hard to believe that one or even a few genes are responsible for all of them. Nevertheless, from the genetic point of view, it is quite possible.

The ability of a gene to influence several phenotypic traits is called pleiotropy. For example, the gene for red hair causes lighter skin color and freckles. A mutation in the gene that codes for the enzyme phenylalanine-4-hydroxylase (which catalyzes the conversion of the amino acid phenylalanine to tyrosine) is the basis of phenylketonuria, a disease characterized by mental retardation, hair loss, and skin pigmentation. The pleiotropy phenomenon can be explained by the fact that the product of virtually every gene is often involved in multiple processes that form the metabolic network of the body. This is especially characteristic of genes encoding signaling proteins facilitating intercellular communication (Larange A., Cheroutre H., 2016).

Retinol is a natural gene regulator, and retinoid receptors are an integral part of the regulatory apparatus of the cellular genome. Although the mechanism of direct action of retinol on the cell is universal, the cell response depends on its type and its role in the skin. It is very likely that different cell types have different sets of retinoid receptors (so far, six variants have been found, but there may be more). Hence, different genes are activated in different cells. Alternatively, it could be that different receptors can bind to the same gene, but their effect is different (for example, some receptors inhibit while others activate gene expression). Both assumptions are plausible but remain at the level of hypotheses.

4.2. Dermal effects of retinoids

The effects of retinol on the skin have been compared to an iceberg: we only see the tip — the clinical effects, which are the result of changes in the cells deep within the skin (Kang S., 2005; Riahi R.R. et al., 2016). To understand the visible effects of retinol, it is important to remember that retinol acts only on living cells, with different cell types responding differently. In the case of skin, the following picture emerges (**Table II-4-1**).

The action of retinol on the cell can be not only direct, i.e., through the nuclear receptors, but also indirect, which can be likened to a game of skittles. It is not necessary for the ball to hit all the pins at once: it is enough to hit one successfully, and the others start falling, knocking each other down. In the same way, when retinol gets into a cell, it stimulates the production of biologically active substances (cytokines), which are released into the intercellular space and, in turn, act on other cells.

Retinoids are small, lipophilic molecules that easily penetrate the *stratum corneum*. We can say that the *stratum corneum* is transparent for them. They just as easily penetrate the greasy hair follicles. A retinoid concentration gradient is created in the skin, decreasing towards the dermis. In the epidermis, retinoids control keratinization and pigmentation processes. In the dermal layer, they restore the intercellular matrix gradually degraded in the process of aging or UV exposure. The transfollicular pathway makes it possible to obtain an increased concentration of retinoids directly in the follicles, which is especially valuable in treating follicular pathologies, including acne.

In the scientific and medical literature, many articles are published each year on the effects of retinoids on the skin, both desirable and

Table II-4-1. Effects of retinoids on the skin at different levels

LEVEL	DESCRIPTION
Clinical	- Visible scaling - Skin lightening - Smoothing wrinkles - Accelerated wound healing - Improved skin firmness and elasticity - Irritation
Histological	- Thinning of the *stratum corneum* - Thickening of the living layers of the epidermis - Changing the structure of the dermis (collagen matrix)
Cellular	- Stimulation of basal keratinocyte proliferation - Stimulation of fibroblasts to the synthesis of intercellular matrix components - Suppression of secretory activity of sebocytes
Immunological	- Stimulation of Langerhans cells to present antigens - Induction of keratinocyte expression of intercellular adhesive molecules that play an important role in intercellular communication and development of immune response - Modulation of production of some cytokines, including those involved in inflammatory and immune reactions
Biochemical	- Regulation of keratinocyte differentiation (in particular, influence on keratin and involucrin expression) - Regulation of the activity of enzymes involved in melanin synthesis - Reduction of keratinocyte production of vascular endothelial growth factor, which affects the development of blood capillaries in the skin - Regulation of lipid and keratin synthesis in sebocytes - Reducing the level and activity of dermal metalloproteinases and connective tissue enzymes that degrade the intercellular matrix
Molecular	- Effect on the level of intracellular retinoic acid binding proteins - Activation of gene expression through nuclear receptors (RARs and RXRs)

undesirable (Khalil S. et al., 2017). We have selected what we believe to be the most interesting facts, paying special attention to those that have direct implications for practical dermatology (**Table II-4-2**).

Table II-4-2. Main cellular targets of retinol in the skin responsible for clinical outcome

TARGET CELL	CELLULAR RESPONSE	CHANGES IN THE SKIN TISSUE	CLINICAL OUTCOME
Keratinocyte	• Stimulation of division, maturation, and migration	• Updating the cellular composition of the epidermis • Thinning of the *stratum corneum*	• Smoothing of microrelief, reduction of keratosis signs • Reducing the expression of wrinkles • Tone leveling • In case of an excessive dose — dryness of the *stratum corneum*
Sebocyte	• Suppression of sebum production	• Reducing the amount of sebum • Normalization of the sebum composition	• Reducing oily shine
Fibroblast	• Stimulation of synthetic activity	• Changes in the structure of the intercellular matrix: improvement of the collagen–elastin framework	• Improved skin elasticity and turgor • Smoothing fine lines and wrinkles
Langerhans cell	• Modulation of the ability to present antigen • Reduced production of inflammatory mediators in keratinocytes	• Restoration of vascular wall permeability • Reduction of tissue infiltration by immunocytes	• Reduction of erythema • Reduction of local edema

4.2.1. Keratinocytes and keratinization of the epidermis

Retinoids affect the proliferation and differentiation of basal keratinocytes, accelerating epidermal renewal (Fisher C. et al., 1995; Li J. et al., 2019). The full picture of their action is not completely clear, but some aspects are already known. For example, retinoids inhibit the expression of the gene encoding type VII collagen, the main component of the "anchoring" fibrils that ensure the adhesion of corneocytes to the basal membrane. As a result, the connection of cells to the basal membrane is weakened. They more quickly detach from it and start to move upwards (Törmä H., 2011).

Detachment from the basal membrane is regarded as a trigger signal for differentiation, which is most closely related to keratin synthesis. Although the cell detached from the basal membrane no longer divides, it is still alive and has active metabolic processes underlying the transformation of a keratinocyte into a corneocyte.

Thus, basal keratinocytes differ significantly in their keratin profile from the overlying cells. It is known that the family of keratin proteins includes many varieties (Virtanen M. et al., 2001), which replace each other during keratinocyte transformation into a corneocyte. This process is under the control of several mediators, including keratinocyte growth factor, epidermal growth factor, retinoids, and calcium. Experiments on human keratinocyte culture have shown that the morphological picture rapidly changes if retinol is removed from the culture medium. The number of cells with signs of complete keratinization increases (which is manifested by changes in their keratin profile and appearance of 1/10 and 6/16 keratin pairs characteristic of horny scales), their adhesion to each other increases, and their motility decreases.

Another distinctive feature of corneocytes is the presence of a rigid protein−lipid shell called the cornified envelope. The synthesis of the involucrin protein, which is part of the cornified envelope, is also controlled by retinoids in the process of keratinocyte differentiation.

Interestingly, *trans*-RA at concentrations of about 10^{-6} M suppresses keratinocyte proliferation, while enhancing it at lower concentrations (about 10^{-7} M). A similar effect is observed in the case of glandular epithelium, including sebaceous gland cells, and is explained by the activation of different receptor types.

Through keratinocytes, retinoids also affect other skin cells. For example, retinol reduces the production and release by normal keratinocytes of growth factors of epithelial cells lining blood capillaries, thus preventing excessive development of the capillary network. Moreover, retinol induces expression by keratinocytes of glycoproteins and type I intercellular adhesive molecules, which play an important role in intercellular communication and the immune cascade development.

4.2.2. Sebocytes and acne

Vitamin A is one of the regulators of sebaceous glands and is necessary for their normal functioning.

Lipid and keratin synthesis are two important aspects, as well as indicators of sebocyte activity. One of the first successful studies devoted to this topic was published several years after the discovery of retinoid receptors — in 1991 (Zouboulis C. C. et al., 1991). Three retinoids were considered: natural *trans*-RA and synthetic 13-*cis*-retinoic acid (13-*cis*-RA, or isotretinoin) and acitretin. It turned out that the severity of the effect largely depends on the chemical structure of the retinoid. Thus, 13-*cis*-RA exhibited the strongest inhibitory effect on lipid synthesis (48.2%), followed by *trans*-RA (38.6%) and acitretin (27.5%). All retinoids significantly inhibit the synthesis of triglycerides, fatty esters and waxes, and fatty acids in sebocytes; at the same time, squalene synthesis remains unchanged, and cholesterol synthesis is even slightly activated.

The situation is also ambiguous for keratin. The result depends on the nature of the retinoid and its concentration, as well as the type of keratin. Accordingly, retinoids suppress keratin-5 synthesis and have almost no effect on keratin-13. Keratin-6 and -16 are suppressed by both 13-*cis*-RA and *trans*-RA, while keratin-14 is suppressed only by 13-*cis*-RA. At the same time, *trans*-RA increases keratin-19 synthesis. Acitretin has no pronounced effect on keratinization.

The main conclusion is that local vitamin A deficiency can lead to the development of acne disease, characterized by impaired synthetic processes in sebocytes and increased cell proliferation. This is confirmed by the efficacy of the topical application of trans-RA (tretinoin preparations) in mild to moderate acne, which compensates for retinoid deficiency.

There are situations when, for some reason, the rate of *trans*-RA inactivation increases in sebocytes, resulting in a lower-than-normal intracellular concentration. This occurs, for example, with some mutations in cytochrome P_{450}. Cytochrome P_{450} is involved in the intracellular transformation of retinol and natural retinoids. When cytochrome P_{450} activity is increased, the concentration of active retinoids in the cell decreases, and patients show all the signs of acne — abnormal sebocytes and hyperkeratinization of the sebaceous gland duct. In such cases, the use of synthetic retinoids that are more resistant to intracellular transformations and yet capable of activating RAR receptors may be even more effective than natural retinoids (Kim M.J. et al., 2000).

Isotretinoin is traditionally used to treat severe acne and seborrhea. Systemic therapy with isotretinoin leads to a decrease in the size of sebaceous glands (by almost 90%) owing to suppression of proliferation and differentiation of basal sebocytes and inhibition of lipid synthesis (by 75%).

Tripharotene is a new topical retinoid for the treatment of acne, which appeared on the market in 2019 (see Part II, section 4.1.3). It is highly specific to RAR-γ and has shown a good safety profile in addition to its proven efficacy in clinical trials in the treatment of acne (Aubert J. et al., 2018; Scott L.J., 2019).

4.2.3. Hair follicle cells and hair loss

Hair follicle cells are another type of skin epithelial cells. Of particular interest are the cells concentrated in the bulge area. This area is located on the side in the upper part of the follicle in the form of a small protrusion (bulge). It is believed that this is where the stem cells are located, which proliferate in the early anagen stage, gradually shifting to the lower part of the follicle. Upon reaching the papilla, they begin to differentiate, acquiring the features of keratinocytes involved in constructing the hair shaft. When the area adjacent to the follicle is damaged, the bulge acts as a donor of stem cells, which take part in restoring the skin.

It is not yet clear whether retinoids directly affect proliferation, i.e., reproduction of stem cells, but they control the process of differentiation, as evidenced by several experiments (Lu Z. et al., 2020; VanBuren C.A., Everts H.B., 2022). Retinoids can also indirectly affect hair growth by stimulating the development of microcapillaries and improving the blood supply to the papilla.

So far, all attempts to use retinoids to treat alopecia have failed to yield significant results, but their combination with minoxidil seems quite successful and increases the effectiveness of treatment compared to the use of minoxidil alone (Sharma A. et al., 2019). Nevertheless, this area of retinoid use remains poorly understood, and it is too early to draw any definite conclusions.

4.2.4. Langerhans cells and skin immunity

Langerhans cells (skin macrophages), the only immune cells in the epidermis, are also sensitive to retinol. Macrophages recognize a foreign agent (antigen), capture it, and then produce an antibody. After leaving the epidermis and penetrating local lymph nodes, macrophages present the antigen to T-lymphocytes, which can recognize it on their own the next time they encounter the antibody. As it turned out, retinol modulates the ability of macrophages to present the antigen (Meunier L. et al., 1994).

At the same time, the functions of Langerhans cells in the epidermis are much wider than the control of "outsiders." Activated macrophages produce many biologically active substances affecting the microenvironment and participating in the maintenance of local homeostasis. Among them are important regulators of the inflammatory process, such as IL-1β, TNF-α, and nitric oxide (NO). The release of these substances was also found to be controlled by retinoic acid. Thus, retinoic acid inhibits macrophage production of NO, prevents subsequent accumulation of nitrites in the intercellular medium, and lowers the levels of TNF-α and IL-1β. These data to some extent explain the anti-inflammatory effect of *trans*-RA (Oliveira L. M. et al., 2018), which, in particular, is one of the prerequisites for the use of retinoids in the treatment of psoriasis.

4.2.5. Melanocytes and skin pigmentation

A mild whitening effect usually accompanies the use of retinoids. This indicates that retinoids interfere with skin pigmentation processes.

While how this happens is still not entirely clear, a number of studies have shown that retinoic acid affects the activity of tyrosinase, a key enzyme of melanin synthesis. Some researchers note a suppression of tyrosinase activity in the presence of retinoids, especially in UV-irradiated skin, while others, on the contrary, report an increase in it. Interestingly, tyrosinase activation is characteristic only for white skin, while retinoic acid does not affect tyrosinase activity in black skin.

Researchers are unanimous in the opinion that tyrosinase activity regulation occurs not due to the effect of *trans*-RA on the expression of the gene encoding the enzyme itself but as a result of some not yet fully understood post-transcriptional mechanisms. In other words, the effect of *trans*-RA on the working enzyme is already evident.

Retinoic acid can also directly affect melanocytes through the receptor apparatus. A retinoic acid-binding protein, CRABP-I, was found in melanocytes, but its transition into the active form depends not only on the presence of *trans*-RA. It turned out that the ability of CRABP-I to bind *trans*-RA is largely determined by the cellular environment — keratinocytes and fibroblasts; in contrast, CRABP-I of isolated melanocytes has low activity. Here we again encounter an example of the exceptional role of intercellular interactions: skin cells are members of a single community, determining each other's behavior (Lu Z. et al., 2020).

The importance of retinoic regulation for melanocytes can be illustrated by additional interesting facts (Coleman D. J., 2014). For example, as human melanoma progresses, RXRα type II receptor expression is lost, leading to the uncontrolled proliferation of melanocytes.

It has also been demonstrated that, after acute UV irradiation, melanocytes of mice with melanocyte-specific ablation of genes encoding RXRα and RXRβ attract fewer interferon γ-secreting immune cells than melanocytes of wild-type mice. This is because defective melanocytes have decreased the production of some chemokines that attract immune cells. As a result, the interferon levels in their microenvironment decline. Against this background, cell apoptosis mechanisms are activated, and the fibroblast survival rate after UV irradiation decreases. Thus, it turns out that RXRα and RXRβ receptors in melanocytes mediate the survival of skin fibroblasts (Coleman D.J., 2014).

4.2.6. Fibroblasts and wrinkle smoothing

The gradual thinning of the dermal layer of the skin during aging (including photoaging) is associated with two parallel processes:
1. Activation of metalloproteinases — intercellular enzymes destroying collagen and elastin fibers of derma
2. Slowing down the synthesis of new collagen by fibroblasts

As a result of the degradation of the dermic intercellular substance, skin elasticity and firmness are reduced, and wrinkles are formed. The use of topical retinoids affects the synthetic activity of fibroblasts and reduces the activity of collagen-degrading metalloproteinases. This experimental finding does not yet have an exact explanation. There may be an indirect effect on fibroblasts through cytokines released by epidermal cells in response to retinoids.

One of the histological signs of skin photodamage is the appearance of abnormal elastin material, which replaces collagen. It has been shown that, after UVB irradiation, the expression of the elastin gene increases several times. Tretinoin applied to irradiated skin acts oppositely — it inhibits the expression of the elastin gene, thus preventing the subsequent synthesis of the protein. Several studies have also shown that retinoids enhance the synthesis of another important matrix component — glycosaminoglycans (Shao Y. et al., 2017). However, this effect is mostly attributed to the mediated effect of retinoid-activated keratinocytes and endothelial cells on fibroblasts during regular use of retinol-containing cosmetic care products.

4.3. Topical retinoids in cosmetic dermatology and skincare

The era of retinoids in dermatology was ushered in by Albert Kligman. In the 1960s, interested in the dermatological effects of *trans*-RA (tretinoin), Kligman discovered its positive effect on acne-prone skin. The first company to market a topical product with retinoic acid was Ortho Pharmaceutical, a subsidiary of Johnson & Johnson. It acquired a patent from Albert Kligman, and in 1971 the Retin-A (0.1% tretinoin) acne treatment was introduced to the general public and quickly gained popularity. Twenty-five years later, in 1996, Ortho Pharmaceutical launched another remedy, Renova, designed to prevent skin changes due to aging and promote repair after photodamage. Renova contains 0.05% tretinoin encased in a soft cream base and is used to combat fine lines and hyperpigmentation. Renova was the first photoaging drug to receive FDA approval.

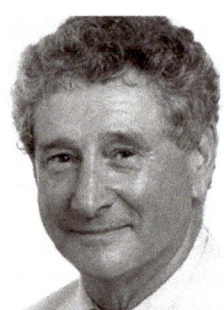

Albert Kligman
(1916–2010)

Consumers appreciated retinoin preparations, and other pharmaceutical companies followed the successful example of Ortho Pharmaceutical (albeit with great caution). Both Retin-A and Renova, as well as generics containing tretinoin, are considered medicines. Accordingly, they must have medical registration, be sold in pharmacies, and be prescribed by doctors.

In the mid-1990s, cosmetics with vitamin A appeared, and the indications for their use were almost the same: oily skin, acne, and photoaging. The range of cosmetic products with retinol offered today is quite broad — from face creams to nail care products. Here are the main categories of retinol cosmetics:
1. Skincare products:
   - Rejuvenation (prevention and treatment of age-related skin changes and photoaging)
   - Sebum control (for oily skin)
   - Acne-prone skin
   - Post-acne

2. After-sun cosmetics (for prevention of photodamage)
3. Nail care products
4. Peel products

There are even sunscreens with retinol, though it is not quite clear why they contain retinol — when exposed to direct sunlight, all its activity immediately disappears. It is much more reasonable to use retinol in cosmetics after sunburn and in night nourishing and regenerating creams in which the normalizing qualities of vitamin A are essential.

4.3.1. Drugs and cosmetic formulations

Several questions are addressed here, including: How should retinoid-based topical products be classified? Why do some have medical registration with all the ensuing requirements for sale and prescription, while others are sold uncontrolled and classified as cosmetics?

To begin with, all synthetic retinoids are medicinal substances and are not approved for use in cosmetics.

As for natural retinoids (endogenous derivatives of vitamin A), it all depends on their form:
- Biologically active *trans*-RA or 13-*cis*-RA are drug substances.
- Precursors (retinol, retinal, retinyl esters) are cosmetic ingredients.

Recall that cells store retinol and convert it into the active form as needed, which binds to nuclear receptors. If the cell is "fed" *trans*-RA, it can no longer self-regulate the number of active molecules it needs, and the cellular response is forced, fast, and pronounced. If retinol or its esters get into the cell, they are deposited and then gradually activated, so the effect is slow and not so readily apparent. **Cosmetic products are based on an intracrine concept: precursors are applied to the skin and are transformed into a biologically active form in the skin cells (Fig. II-4-7)**. In this regard, it is more correct to use the terms "retinol skincare products" and "retinoid medication" (**Fig. II-4-8**).

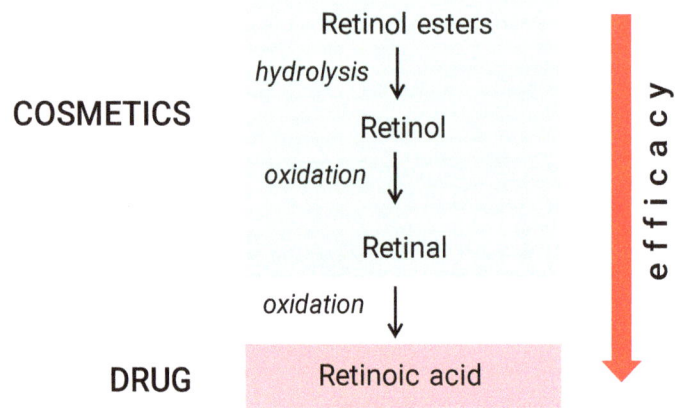

Figure II-4-7. Intracrine concept of retinoid use

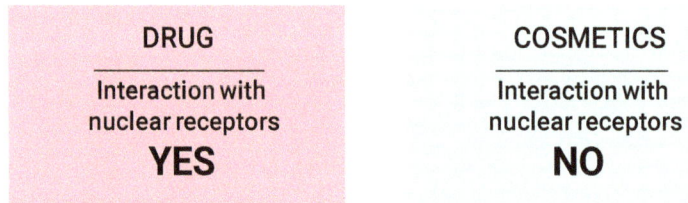

Bioactive forms:
- *trans*-RA (tretinoin)
- 9-*cis*-RA (alitretinoin)
- 13-*cis*-RA (isotretinoin)
- Synthetic retinoids

Inactive forms (precursor or metabolites)
- Retinol esters
- **Retinol (pure vitamin A)**
- Retinal
- Oxoretinoids

Figure II-4-8. Cosmetics or drugs: the principle of retinoid selection

4.3.2. Adverse effects and contraindications to the use of retinol cosmetics

When using retinol cosmetics, skin redness, temporary scaling, rarely blistering, and increased sensitivity to sunlight have been reported in some cases. This should be considered when formulating, and if possible, selecting the components in such a way as to reduce the risk of adverse reactions.

Among the contraindications to retinol cosmetics is the simultaneous use of photosensitizing drugs such as thiazides, tetracyclines, fluoroquinolones, phenothiazines, and sulfonamides.

Products with retinol should not be used for low-sebum dry skin as retinol further reduces sebum secretion.

We would especially like to mention the problem of using retinol cosmetics by pregnant women. Even though the concentration of retinol and/or its esters in cosmetics is low, and it is believed that they are not absorbed into the blood, it is still better to apply caution and refrain from using it during pregnancy and lactation. Remember that vitamin A has a strong teratogenic effect and that retinol drugs are strictly contraindicated for pregnant women.

4.4. Prescription features of retinol products

The kinetics of retinoids in the skin and their physiological activity depend on their chemical structure and therefore vary considerably. The biologically active form of vitamin A *trans*-RA has a rather high irritant potential and is used exclusively for medical purposes for a limited time. Biologically inactive forms — retinol and its esters (retinyl palmitate or retinyl acetate) — are included in cosmetics for mass use.

4.4.1. Choosing the optimal dose

The optimal dose is one at which visible improvements can be expected while eliminating the risk of undesirable effects associated with overdose. Many questions also arise regarding dose selection, the first of which is the permeability of the substance and its accumulation in the various structures of the skin. Retinol penetrates the skin best, followed by retinyl palmitate and retinyl acetate.

The choice of vitamin A concentration and its esters depends on the purpose and objectives of the cosmetic product (**Table II-4-3**). Care preparations are used permanently and are intended for the physiological regulation of skin cells to prevent/treat signs of aging and photoaging and to control sebum production. Peel preparations are single-acting to stimulate exfoliation. In prophylactic products, the retinol concentration is usually lower than average. Products for treating

Table II-4-3. Recommended doses of retinol, retinyl palmitate, and retinyl acetate in cosmetic products (assuming an initial concentration of 1 million IU/g)

RETINOL, %	RETINYL PALMITATE, %	RETINYL ACETATE, %
Day cream.............0.05–0.1 Night cream............0.1–0.2 Hand cream................0.05 Body milk..............0.05–0.1 After-sun cream.....0.1–0.2 After-sun body milk..............0.05–0.1 **Peel mask........... app. 1% (up to 10%)**	Cream/Lotion.....0.1–0.5 Shampoo.............0.1–0.5 Conditioner.........0.1–0.5 Nail care products..............0.1–0.5	Day cream...........0.5–5.0 Night cream........0.5–5.0 Body milk............0.5–2.0 After-sun face cream..................3.0–5.0 After-sun body milk............1.0–3.0

the symptoms of photoaging have higher concentrations. The highest retinol concentration (about 1%) is found in peel products. Sometimes several forms of vitamin A are included in the formulation, for example:
- Retinyl esters + retinol
- Retinyl esters + retinol + retinal

These inactive precursors are at different stages in the chain of conversion to retinoic acid (see **Fig. II-4-2**) and are thus activated at different rates. Using such combinations makes it possible, on the one hand, to increase the total concentration of vitamin A in the formulation and, on the other hand, to ensure its gradual activation and prolong action while maintaining its safety.

4.4.2. How to keep retinol active

Vitamin A is a very unstable substance that rapidly degrades when exposed to light and oxidizes in the air. Vitamin A esters are more stable but flammable and can ignite in the air, so working with them requires great care and careful observance of all rules for storage and handling. Personal safety precautions should also be followed, and the substance should not come into contact with the skin, respiratory or gastrointestinal tract.

It is very difficult to avoid contact with the air in the process of making a cosmetic product. Consequently, some of the vitamin A is inactivated before the product reaches the consumer. To avoid unnecessary losses, special conditions for the manufacture of retinol preparations should be followed. For example, some production steps should be carried out in an inert gas atmosphere.

Vitamin A is added directly into the dehydrated base or oil phase of the cream or lotion at 35–40 °C and even lower temperatures, if possible. Special emulsifiers, such as polysorbate-80, are used in water-based preparations to give the product a homogeneous appearance. The temperature during the entire production cycle should not exceed 45 °C.

It is recommended to introduce antioxidants in the oil phase to prevent oxidation of vitamin A. Vitamin E is the antioxidant of choice because it is also oil-soluble. Vitamin E can be combined with ascorbyl palmitate (a stabilized, oil-soluble form of vitamin C). Over time, cosmetics with retinyl palmitate can turn yellow, and even an antioxidant stabilizer such as butyloxyanisole, with which vitamin A is usually supplied, cannot completely prevent this process. Creams containing vitamins A and E usually do not turn yellow, even if stored at room temperature and occasionally exposed to light.

The water used to make the product should be distilled and deionized, since even trace amounts of metals can cause oxidation of retinyl palmitate. Chelating agents can be used as a safety precaution.

The pH of the finished product must be 5–6 for greater stability. It is best to pack preparations in aluminum tubes or at least in light-tight tubes with a narrow outlet. Some retinol preparations include plant extracts enriched with antioxidants, such as green tea and ginkgo biloba extracts.

Even if all production precautions are observed and vitamin A loss is minimal, the product is exposed to air and light when applied to the skin. Physical UV filters such as titanium dioxide and zinc oxide, which act as reflectors, help to partially prevent vitamin A degradation by UV rays. For this reason, their inclusion into the finished product is also recommended.

The choice of oils should be made very carefully. Do not get carried away with unsaturated oils — vitamin A needs an oxidation-resistant base. Some retinol formulas include shea butter, squalene, lanolin, and even cholesterol. Silicone oils have proven to be quite good as they are not subject to oxidation and, in addition, improve the appearance of the product.

Additional stabilization of retinyl palmitate and an increase in its penetrating power are achieved using some transdermal carriers, such as solid lipid nanoparticles made of glyceryl behenate. The nanoparticle suspension has a low viscosity. In contrast to membrane carriers (e.g., liposomes), these nanoparticles are stable in forms convenient for topical applications, such as hydrogels and oil-in-water emulsions. Glyceryl behenate is very resistant to oxidation since it contains saturated behenic acid. Surrounded by such a coating, retinyl palmitate is reliably protected against oxidation, even during product application and distribution on the skin. Another major advantage of this system is the gradual release of the active ingredient, which prolongs the drug's effect. Studies have shown that most of the nanoparticles remain bound to the skin's surface layers, and retinyl palmitate is released for at least 18 h after application.

Relatively recently, another interesting carrier system for bioactive ingredients has appeared on the cosmetics market — microsponges. These are soft, porous structures made of inert material. They are like a sponge and absorb substances effectively, so they can be loaded with various active agents. Once on the skin, the microsponges remain on the surface and gradually release their contents, especially if they are slightly deformed with a gentle massage. The retinol in the microsponges is protected from direct contact with the air and does not degrade as quickly. The fact that it enters the skin in doses increases its safety and prolongs its action.

4.4.3. Combination with other active substances

For safety reasons, cosmetic products containing vitamin A should not be overloaded with other active ingredients. This applies primarily to those compounds that have a similar effect. Thinning the *stratum corneum* and increasing the proliferation of keratinocytes (α-hydroxy acids, keratolytics, proteolytic enzymes) act as immunomodulators (β-glucans) and regulators of collagen synthesis (phytoestrogens). Vitamin A is a very strong agent, so it is better not to risk turning the drug into a "rattlesnake mixture."

Vitamin A combines well with many vitamins, although the motives for such combinations are different. We mentioned vitamins E and C when discussing ways to preserve vitamin A in the formulation (see Part II, section 4.4.2). The combination of vitamins A and D stimulates epidermal cell growth, regulates granulation, and promotes faster burn healing. Combining the four vitamins A, E, C and D increases the skin's resistance to adverse conditions such as cold and improves the preparation's stability.

4.5. Peculiarities of retinol peeling "within-out"

Retinol-driven scaling is different from scaling by damage to the skin's barrier structures. Retinol does not destroy skin proteins like keratolytics (phenol, TCA, salicylic acid) because it does not react chemically with proteins and amino acids. Retinol does not change the pH within the *stratum corneum* and therefore does not directly affect the activity of enzymes.

The *stratum corneum* is "transparent" for retinol — due to its lipophilicity and small size, retinol molecules easily pass through it without staying long. Dead, nuclear DNA-free corneocytes don't react to retinol, and there is no direct damaging effect on enzymes or other *stratum corneum* components.

Only living cells are sensitive to retinol. They respond by expressing several genes, including those responsible for cell division, which is why rapidly dividing cells are most susceptible to retinoids. In the skin, these cells are basal keratinocytes and sebocytes, so the most striking effects of retinoids on the skin are associated with these cells.

Thus, basal keratinocytes activated by retinoids begin to divide faster and move upward, pushing out the overlying cell layers, which manifests in visible skin scaling. This is why retinol peeling is called an "inside-out" peeling.

At the same time, the rate of keratinocyte maturation (differentiation) lags behind the rate of division (proliferation) and migration. Therefore, unlike fine scaling after glycolic peeling, after retinol peeling large scales are observed (**Fig. II-4-9**), indicating the *stratum corneum*'s immaturity.

In preparations for intensive peel, the retinol concentration is higher than in products for routine skincare. Special creams with up to 10% retinol content are used for professional chemical peeling. Retinol colors the product yellow, so the peel is called Yellow Peel. *trans*-RA (5–10% tretinoin) can also be used instead of retinol, but the product must pass medical registration in this case.

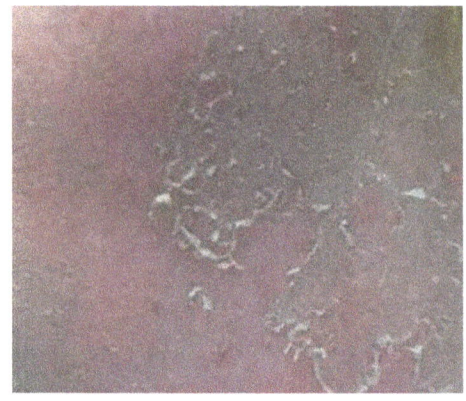

Figure II-4-9. Skin scaling triggered by retinol peel product

In addition to retinol/retinoic acid, salicylic acid (keratolytic) may be present in the peel formulation. These substances combine chemically (both are lipophilic) and biologically (they have different targets and mechanisms of action, and both inhibit sebum production). This combination is justified for peel products. However, it is likely to cause intense scaling and irritation when included in regularly used skincare products.

Phytic, kojic, and azelaic acids, known for their inhibitory effect on melanin synthesis, can often be found in retinol peels. Phytic acid, among its other properties, is a chelator of divalent ions and binds iron ions, thus preventing the development of oxidative stress in the skin. Vitamins, , as well as anti-inflammatory and soothing additives (e.g., chamomile extract, aloe, allantoin, vitamin C, etc.) may be included in the formulation.

4.6. Practical aspects

Indications for retinol peeling:
- Epidermal melasma
- Pigment spots
- Superficial wrinkles
- Oily skin
- Post-acne

Contraindications:
- Low-sebum dry skin
- Taking other vitamin A-containing products (to avoid an overdose)
- Current or history of liver disease
- Injuries and skin scratches in the target area
- Severe acne
- Pregnancy, lactation
- Individual intolerance

The peel procedure is uncomplicated and easily tolerated. The general protocol is as follows. After cleansing, the skin is scrubbed with a lotion with AHAs or salicylic acid in small concentrations to increase the *stratum corneum* permeability and prepare the skin for applying a yellow mask. The mask is applied in a thin, even layer to the whole face or a separate area, left for some time (from 20 minutes to 2 hours, depending on the skin condition and retinol concentration), and then washed off with a cleanser.

Depending on the task, the procedure can be repeated several times at two-hour intervals. For example, in the case of epidermal melasma, it is enough to make 2–3 repeated applications. This provokes a superficial peel with minimal inflammation. To work with wrinkles, photodamaged skin, and the effects of acne, 5–6 applications of four-hour duration may be required. This results in pronounced scaling and more severe inflammation, but the renewal effect is also more noticeable.

After about a day or two, there is a feeling of tightness, and flaking begins on the Day 4–5. After about a week, the skin is smoother and fresher. It looks noticeably better after just one treatment, but for the most pronounced and durable effect, the course must include at least three treatments at intervals of 10–14 days.

In the post-peel period, the skin should be treated with a special protective, restorative preparation (Vaseline or even hydrocortisone ointment is possible) several times a day for 3–5 days until it regains its barrier structures. Attention should also be paid to skin moisturization. After about five days, you can start using bleaching products, but only those that do not contain hydroxy acids, retinol, or proteolytic enzymes. If the procedure is performed in the sunny season, during and after the course of retinol peel, it is necessary to use products with high SPF because the skin with the upper layers removed is very sensitive to pigmentation.

The question regarding the depth of retinol peels is not as clear-cut as it seems at first glance. Many publications state that retinol peels are "superficial." It is difficult to agree with this assertion because retinol targets the basal keratinocytes, which is the level of activity of medium-depth peels.

However, unlike all other peeling agents, retinol acts by stimulating the living cells rather than destroying specific skin structures. Therefore, the skin tolerates the retinol peel procedure easily — there is no pain (sometimes there is a slight tingling sensation, but it is not significant), persistent swelling, or erythema. Severe scaling, which is a consequence of a sharp imbalance between the rate of division of basal keratinocytes and the rate of desquamation, passes fairly quickly. We can thus state that, with retinol peel, it is possible to achieve non-traumatic and complete renewal of the epidermis on all its levels.

> Retinol peels are recommended once or twice a year. The best time is in late fall, winter, and early spring. The retinol peel procedure is a cosmetic procedure and can be performed by a skincare specialist with secondary medical education. Moreover, sometimes patients perform it on their own at home because it is relatively safe.

Part III

General principles of chemical peeling

The protocols of the chemical peeling procedure with different compositions differ in detail. We have written about them in the relevant sections. But there are general points that must be remembered.

1.1. Choice of peel formulation

In modern skincare practice, chemical peels are increasingly seen as an effective way to treat changes that primarily affect the epidermis. In this regard, preference is given to lighter peels. Aesthetic defects resulting from changes in the dermal layer are treated by injections or energy-based physical methods that, due to their minimally invasive nature, do not cause severe damage to the skin's barrier structures and work specifically in the deeper skin layers. Due to this division of "spheres of responsibility," chemical peels are successfully combined with other methods of aesthetic medicine without trying to achieve more than these treatments are capable of (Weissler J.M. et al., 2017).

Regarding the previously widespread opinion that "the more inflammation/injury, the more effective the peel," it is now understood that an inflammatory reaction can be an ally, but only if it is not severe and passes quickly. In the case of severe inflammation and its chronicity, on the contrary, the risk of complications becomes considerably greater. For this reason, preference is increasingly given to more gentle superficial peels. At the stage of post-peeling recovery, particular emphasis is placed on anti-inflammatory measures and additional protection (until the barrier structures of the *stratum corneum* are restored) (O'Connor A.A. et al., 2018).

As for exfoliation, it is indicated at any age. Periodic skin cleansing and removal of surface impurities and scales visibly revitalize the skin and improve its appearance. Delicate enzymatic peels and mechanical exfoliation with a scrub can be done at home as a supportive treatment.

In general, ideal candidates for chemical peels are people with signs of photoaging and early symptoms of natural aging, uneven pigmentation, and keratosis (see Part I, section 1.1). The results are not as impressive with flabbiness, ptosis (deformational aging), and deep wrinkles since the improvement achieved with peels can be lost in changes that peels cannot eliminate. In this case, there is a need to use a combination of minimally invasive injectables (fillers, threads, botulinum toxin therapy, mesotherapy, platelet-rich plasma (PRP) therapy), energy-based (RF lifting, ultrasonic lifting, fractional photolysis, and RF thermolysis) and even surgical (surgical lift) methods (Lee J.C. et al., 2016).

Table III-1-1 provides comparative information on the mechanisms of action and clinical effects of different peeling agents, and the diagram in **Fig. III-1-1** gives an idea of the depth at which the peeling agents work (Starkman S.J., Mangat D.S., 2020).

Table III-1-1. Mechanisms of action and clinical effects of different peeling agents

MECHANISM OF ACTION	MOLECULAR	CELLULAR	HISTO-LOGICAL	CLINICAL
Phenol				
Keratolytic, denaturing and destroying protein structures	Breaks intra- and intermolecular protein disulfide bonds	Damage to extracellular protein structures and cells (up to their death)	Starts the repair of all skin layers through damage to cells and extracellular protein structures	• Scaling of damaged skin • Pain, swelling, erythema • Restructuring of damaged skin tissue • Irreversible impairment of the melanogenesis

Continued on p. 134

MECHANISM OF ACTION	MOLECULAR	CELLULAR	HISTO-LOGICAL	CLINICAL
Trichloracetic acid				
Keratolytic, denaturing and destroying protein structures	Breaks intra- and intermolecular protein disulfide bonds	Damage to extracellular protein structures and cells (up to their death)	Starts the repair of all skin layers through damage to cells and extracellular protein structures	• Scaling of damaged skin • Pain, swelling, erythema (even with medium-depth peels) • Smoothing of microrelief • Lightening and leveling of tone
Salicylic acid				
Keratolytic, denaturing and destroying protein structures	Breaks intra- and intermolecular protein disulfide bonds	• Weakens corneocyte cohesion • Reduces the production of inflammatory mediators	• Loosens the *stratum corneum* • Antiseptic • Reduced sebocyte activity	• Exfoliation of the *stratum corneum* • Alignment of microrelief • Lightening and leveling of skin tone • Reducing sebum production • Reducing inflammation
AHAs, PHAs				
Changes in the pH of the intercellular medium (acidification) of the *stratum corneum* and the living layers of the epidermis	A change in pH modifies the activity of the enzymes of the *stratum corneum*, as a result, the keratinization process is temporarily disrupted	• Increased mitotic activity of basal keratinocytes • Increased number of lamellar bodies in granular keratinocytes	• Accelerating the renewal of the epidermis • Thinning of the *stratum corneum* • Strengthening the barrier of the *stratum corneum*	• Exfoliation of the *stratum corneum* • Alignment of microrelief • Lightening and leveling of skin tone

Continued on p. 135

End of Table III-1-1

MECHANISM OF ACTION	MOLECULAR	CELLULAR	HISTO-LOGICAL	CLINICAL
Proteolytic enzymes				
Weaken the cohesion of corneocytes	Selectively destroy corneodesmosomes as well as protein–lipid contaminants on the skin surface	No effect on living cells	Stimulate cell renewal of the epidermis by accelerating desquamation	• Skin cleansing • Exfoliation of the *stratum corneum* • Alignment of microrelief
Retinol				
Controls proliferation of all living cells; the cells with the highest sensitivity to retinol are rapidly dividing cells	Affects the genetic apparatus of living cells through specific nuclear receptors	Regulates the activity of many genes of all skin cell types, including: • keratinocyte genes responsible for cell division, maturation, and migration • Sebocyte genes responsible for sebum production	• Accelerates the processes of cellular renewal of the epidermis • Suppresses the activity of sebum production	• Skin exfoliation • Smoothing of microrelief • Normalization of sebum production

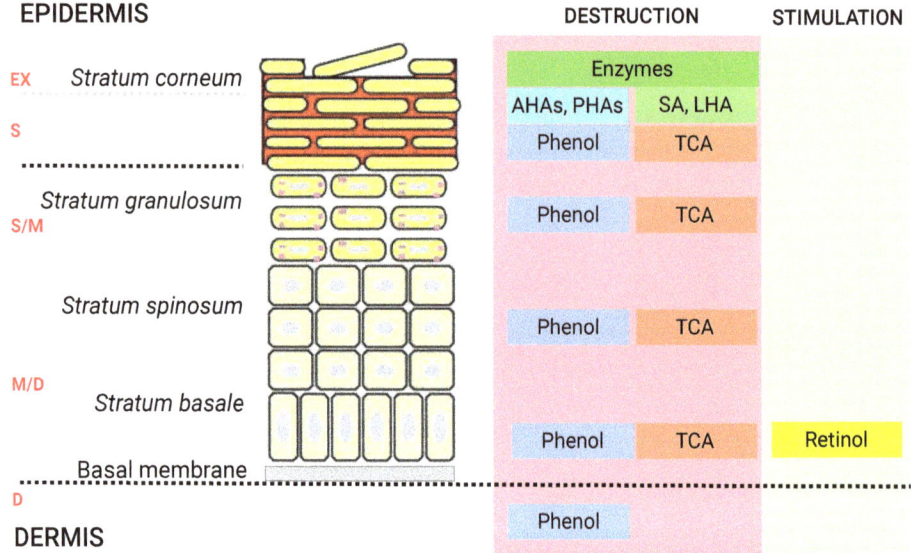

Figure III-1-1. Depth of exposure for different peeling agents

Abbreviations: EX — exfoliation, S — superficial peeling, S/M — superficial/medium-depth peeling, M/D — medium-depth/deep peeling, D — deep peeling, AHAs — α-hydroxy acids, PHAs — polyhydroxy acids, SA — salicylic acid, LHA — lipohydroxy acid

Table III-1-2 classifies the chemical peels according to the depth/degree of damage. Retinol is not in this table because it acts through stimulation of basal keratinocytes rather than through destruction. Its targets are deep, but there is no trauma to the skin.

1.2. Pre-peeling

Skin exfoliation with light acid peels (pH ≈ 3) and enzymatic peels can be done without preparation. Moreover, along with nutraceuticals, it can be an element of pre-peeling skin preparation, which usually begins 1–2 weeks before the procedure.

Proper skin preparation and subsequent restorative care are essential for more aggressive exposures. Direct sunlight should be avoided before and after the chemical peeling (Truchuelo M. et al., 2017).

Table III-1-2. Classification of chemical peels according to the depth of exposure

SKIN LAYER	PEELING AGENTS	INDICATIONS	RECOVERY TIME
Exfoliation (very superficial)			
Stratum corneum	• Enzymes • AHAs (10–20%), pH 3.5–4.5	Uneven pigmentation, slight signs of photoaging, fine surface wrinkles, dull complexion	Quick recovery, scaling is almost invisible
Superficial			
Stratum corneum, granular layer	• AHAs (20–30%), pH 2.5–3.5 • Jessner's solution • Resorcinol (20–30%) • TCA (10%)	Uneven pigmentation, melasma, minor signs of photoaging, fine surface wrinkles	Quick recovery, scaling is almost invisible
Superficial / Medium-depth			
Stratum corneum, granular layer, spiky layer	• Glycolic acid (50–70%), pH 2.0–3.0 • Salicylic acid • Jessner's solution (longer exposure) • Resorcinol (30–50%) • TCA (10–30%)	Hyperpigmentation, melasma, acne, moderate photoaging, wrinkles	Recovery within 1–2 days, more pronounced scaling
Deep / Medium-depth			
All the way down to the basal layer	• Glycolic acid (70%), pH < 1.0 • TCA (up to 50%)	Moderate photoaging, deep wrinkles	About 7 days are needed to heal, redness, some swelling, noticeable scaling
Deep			
Papillary and reticular dermis	• Phenol (88%) • Baker–Gordon's phenol-containing formula	Deep wrinkles, severe photoaging	Healing takes 2–3 weeks. Complications: redness, hyper- or hypopigmentation, infection, scarring

The main goals of pre-peeling preparation of the skin:
- Strengthen its reparative potential
- Weaken the barrier properties of the *stratum corneum*
- Even out the skin microrelief so that the peeling agents penetrate the skin more evenly during the procedure
- Reduce melanocyte activity to avoid the risk of post-inflammatory pigmentation
- Extinguish inflammation (if there is any)

Preparations and ingredients used for pre-peeling preparation:
- AHAs up to 20% and pH not lower than 3.0
- Retinol of about 0.02% to weaken skin barrier properties and thereby reduce the exposure time and concentration of the peeling preparation
- Calcium ion chelators (e.g., phytic acid and EDTA) to reduce corneocyte cohesion
- Depigmenting agents to control the formation of melanin in the skin
- Antioxidants and anti-inflammatory agents

1.3. Peeling procedure

1.3.1. Skin cleansing

Before applying the peeling product, the skin is thoroughly cleansed. The choice of a cleansing solution is important because grease and dirt must be removed without irritating or damaging the skin.

It is, therefore, recommended to use special foams (mousses) based on mild dermatological surfactants rather than alcohol-based solutions.

Modern professional cosmetic brands offer a wide range of cleansers based on synthetic surfactants. These products are balanced in pH. On average, the pH range in this category of products is 4.0–5.5. The choice for each patient is made considering their skin condition, paying attention to:
- Sebum production
- Degree of dryness/humidity of the skin

- Presence/absence of keratosis
- Presence/absence of makeup

In general, when choosing a cleanser, you can follow manufacturer's recommendations. The cleanser should be removed along with the impurities using sponges moistened with warm water. Under no circumstances should it be actively rubbed into the skin. Even if the skin is heavily soiled, it is better to soap a few times with light massaging movements and rinse quickly with water than to "rub" the product into the skin together with the impurities and surfactants.

Before enzymatic and acid peels, after cleansing, the skin should be wiped with a special moisturizing solution to saturate the *stratum corneum* with water. This is necessary because AHAs are water-soluble substances and pass through the hydrated *stratum corneum* faster. Enzymes do not need to pass through the *stratum corneum*, and water is required to promote their proteolytic activity.

Conversely, in case of keratolytic and retinol peels, there is no need to moisturize the skin because these peeling agents are oil-soluble substances, and excess water in the *stratum corneum* only weakens their action.

1.3.2. During the procedure

The peeling preparation is usually applied with a special brush (**Fig. III-1-2**). Beauticians must wear gloves to avoid irritating the skin on their hands. Some time after the application, the patient may have unpleasant sensations — burning (in the case of acid peels), pain

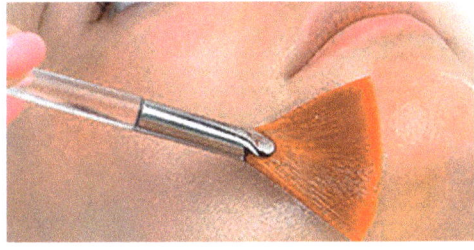

Figure III-1-2. Application of the peel with a brush

(in the case of keratolytics), and tingling (caused by any peel if applied to hypersensitive skin). These are signals that the peel's components have penetrated beneath the *stratum corneum* and are in the living layers of the epidermis. If the discomfort becomes overwhelming, the peeling agent should be immediately removed/washed off or neutralized (in the case of acidic peels). In the case of keratolytic peels, the penetration depth is controlled by frost.

After removing the peeling agent, a soothing agent is applied to the skin, usually a light emulsion with moisturizing and antioxidant components. The procedure is completed with the application of a protective agent. If the peeling is done in the daytime and the patient might spend some time outside after the procedure, the protective product must have UV filters. If there is no risk of sunlight hitting the skin, a thick cream with occlusive properties will suffice. On the one hand, it prevents skin contact with external dust, and on the other hand, it prevents water evaporation, which increases sharply after the impact of peeling products on the *stratum corneum*. The more severe the damage, the more occlusive the product should be.

1.4. Post-treatment rehabilitation

Chemical peeling is an umbrella term for the controlled skin damage methods that are inevitably accompanied by partial or complete destruction of the protective barrier. Thus, it must be appreciated that the increased alertness of skin cells combined with a weakened or even destroyed barrier creates an explosive situation.

The following **undesirable phenomena** may occur immediately after the procedure:
- Itching
- Burning
- Redness
- Edema
- Eye irritation, lacrimation

After a few days, weeks, or even in the longer term, **complications** are possible:
- Infection against the background of a compromised barrier — especially in people with a weak immunity and/or endocrine disorders

- Acne-like lesions — teenagers, mentally unstable people
- Dyschromia (hyper-, hypopigmentation) — people with genetically dark skin (increased basic melanocyte activity) are at risk
- Scarring, delayed healing, skin texture disorders — people with endocrine disorders, adhering to diet restrictions, after an illness

As the skin's defenses are weakened even after superficial peeling, immediately after the procedure and in the early post-peel stage of recovery, the aim is to:
1. Minimize the effect of aggressive external factors and water evaporation by creating an artificial barrier on the skin — UV protection, occlusion
2. Keep the inflammatory process under control, use anti-inflammatory and soothing agents

During the rehabilitation period, corneotherapeutical formulations and non-contact physical therapy treatments with anti-inflammatory effects, such as low-level red and infrared laser therapy (LLLT), are best suited.

1.4.1. Calming agents and inflammation

After superficial peeling, there should be no inflammation, but after medium-depth peeling, it definitely occurs, because living cells are damaged, some of them irreversibly. The inflammatory reaction is the first stage of regeneration, so it cannot be blocked completely. But it is necessary to take measures so that the inflammation is not too strong and does not lead to undesirable consequences.

In skincare practice, substances are used to control the local inflammatory response that modulates inflammation — to modify the processes so that the damage is minimized.

For example, free radicals play a major role in any inflammation. In particular, some immune system cells produce hydrogen peroxide and other ROS to fight infection, which can provoke a cascade of free-radical oxidation reactions in the skin. Therefore, to prevent excessive tissue damage during inflammation, the skin's own antioxidant system can be "strengthened" with cosmetic antioxidants such as **vitamins C and E**, **plant polyphenols**, and **carotenoids**.

Other substances change the set of signaling molecules that cells produce during inflammation. They do this by slightly modifying the direction of chemical processes. This group includes primarily **oils rich in essential fatty acids (omega-3)**. These compounds are precursors of immune system regulatory molecules — prostaglandins — as well as substances of plant origin that inhibit the enzyme's activity responsible for collagen degradation (metalloproteinases), production of inflammatory cytokines, and nitric oxide production, which is also an important participant in inflammatory processes. The difference between such natural substances and medications is that they act gently and, in most cases, do not affect other physiological processes in healthy skin.

The protective barrier of the skin is broken after peeling. Only compositions that do not contain potential irritants and destroyers can be applied to the skin. It can be a soothing gel mask based on polysaccharides, containing **extracts of plants** known in folk medicine or used in food, such as chamomile, aloe, calendula, and plantain. Based on the arsenal of Oriental medicine, we should highlight the Asian centella (gotu-cola). Its aqueous extract contains substances called asiaticosides. They improve epithelialization and reduce inflammation due to immunomodulatory activity.

Purified plant polysaccharides such as **aloe vera polysaccharides, β-glucans, and fucoidans of brown seaweed** have anti-inflammatory and immunomodulatory activity. Brown seaweed fucoidans not only regulate the inflammatory response, which has been shown in allergic skin models, but also stimulate skin renewal processes by increasing the production of collagen, elastin, and glycosaminoglycans, making them an ideal anti-inflammatory ingredient in post-peeling care products. Formulations containing an effective concentration of one, two, or three plants work better and are less likely to cause skin irritation than formulations containing many different extracts.

Warning! Essential oils should be avoided, as many of them are potential allergens and skin irritants. Cooling the skin (with cold compresses or ice) also helps to soothe it.

1.4.2. Occlusive agents and barrier function

Care must be taken to prevent excessive water loss in all cases where the skin's protective barrier is damaged. The greater the damage, the faster the skin must be protected. Otherwise, too intense water evaporation will provoke the release of inflammatory mediators, leading to itching, redness, and swelling, and can subsequently cause hyperpigmentation. Therefore, products with the occlusive effect are necessary after the medium-depth peeling — they allow you to quickly "calm" the skin and prevent the development of the inflammatory reaction in response to the sudden destruction of the barrier structures. Later, it is possible to start using agents that help to restore the barrier, but in those first minutes and hours after the peeling, the priority is to create a protective coating on the skin surface, reducing the evaporation of water. Vaseline-based occlusive ointments are used for this purpose, as they are biologically inert, cope well with their task, and have a long history of use. The ointments may contain anesthetic additives. More modern coatings contain special silicones instead of petroleum jelly. Their advantage is a more comfortable feeling while they are on the skin.

In the case of superficial peeling not accompanied by significant damage to the barrier, a moisturizing cream with aloe gel, hyaluronic acid, and other natural polymers will usually suffice. In this case, it is not necessary to achieve complete occlusion as the main objective is to make sure that the skin does not lose moisture and is not exposed to potential irritants.

At this stage, lamellar and liposomal emulsion-based products are useful. Their composition can include physiological lipids necessary for faster restoration of the skin's lipid barrier — ceramides, unsaturated fatty acids, and cholesterol.

1.4.3. UV filters and sun protection

After chemical peeling, you have to forget about sunbathing for a while. The skin, "opened" during the cosmetic procedure and on full alert, reacts to UV radiation with a sharp increase in melanocyte activity, which can lead to unwanted pigmentation. Ingredients such as AHAs directly increase the skin's sensitivity to UV radiation, which should always be borne in mind.

When choosing a sunscreen, both phototype and the specifics of skincare routine should be considered. For example, if we were talking about a trip to the sea, we would say that dark skin has enough levels of melanin, and using products with high SPF for this skin is unjustified. However, in the case of skin protection after chemical peels, the opposite is true. It is established that melanocytes react not only to UV radiation but also to the appearance of ROS and inflammatory mediators in the skin. Any damage to keratinocytes can lead to melanocyte activation. Since dark skin has been formed under conditions of constant exposure to intense UV radiation, heat, and drastic fluctuations in humidity (from dry to rainy seasons), its melanocytes not only produce large amounts of pigment but also have a more rapid response to activating triggers — UV radiation, ROS, and inflammatory mediators. Accordingly, the risk of hyperpigmentation in such skin is very high. After chemical peels, laser resurfacing, and dermabrasion, patients with dark skin are advised to avoid the sun.

For people with fair and sensitive skin, it is very important that the sunscreen does not irritate the skin. The higher the SPF, the higher the concentration of UV filters, so caution should be exercised here. In most cases, applying sunscreens with SPF 15–30, while avoiding the sun wherever possible, is perfectly adequate. SPF 50+ should only be used when there is a risk of high doses of UV light on the skin. Physical UV filters are thought to have lower irritant potential, so they are preferred.

Since no sunscreen can completely protect the skin from damage, it should be explained to the patient that the sun should be avoided during the skin recovery period. Sunscreens minimize the risk but do not eliminate it.

Sunscreen applied after a cosmetic procedure should be easy to spread, not sticky, not leave a greasy sheen, and not irritate the skin. One way to solve this problem is to use a daytime moisturizer with an SPF of about 15 in combination with a mineral powder containing UV filters. Modern mineral powders have a thin, lightweight texture and usually contain titanium dioxide and/or zinc oxide. This double protection makes it possible to do with a minimal amount of UV filters in the cream, which reduces the risk of skin irritation.

1.5. Influence of nutrition on the clinical effect of chemical peeling

A balanced diet provides the basis for overall health and adequate stress tolerance of the body to various external and internal threats. The most important aspect of stress tolerance is the ability to recover from injury. Healthy skin with normal recovery potential heals quickly and properly. It is important to keep this in mind whenever a cosmetic procedure is contemplated in which the skin will be injured.

It is worth clarifying the patient's food preferences and habits at the planning stage. Virtually any diet that a person follows for ideological or medical reasons limits the intake of certain substances in the body and thus creates the prerequisites for a nutrient imbalance. This imbalance can be prevented or compensated by taking special nutraceuticals, ensuring that the skin receives the substances it needs.

It is well known that nutrition is a powerful epigenetic factor regulating the processes of skin healing and repair (Saldanha S. et al., 2015). There are many different nutraceuticals on the market with different compositions and mechanisms of action. Among the most popular nutraceuticals are amino acids, protein hydrolysates, vitamins, minerals, plant bioflavonoids, hyaluronic acid, and lipids. Which nutraceuticals should be used and when? To answer this question, we need proven facts. Research in this direction is already underway, and the results allow us to draw conclusions and make practical recommendations (Palmieri B. et al., 2019).

1.5.1. Pre-peeling preparation

Before peeling, it is recommended to raise the level of total antioxidants in the body — this is seen as an effective prevention of oxidative stress and post-inflammatory pigmentation. To do this, include plenty of fruits and vegetables in your diet and/or take nutraceuticals with vitamin C and plant bioflavonoids (centella, ginkgo biloba). Probiotics and omega-3 unsaturated fatty acids can help improve immune status and reduce skin reactivity.

1.5.2. Rehabilitation

After a chemical peeling, both respiratory and metabolic processes are activated in the skin cells. During this period, skin needs substances that help the cells maintain energy resources at the necessary level and substances that represent building material. The first group includes coenzyme Q and NADH, which are essential for mitochondrial function. The second group includes substances such as:

- Amino acids — the skin's proteins are built from them, and some of them — arginine, proline and hydroxyproline, N-acetylcysteine and glutamine — have shown to be physiological regulators of the healing
- Micronutrients — many are coenzymes, but researchers have noted a special role for zinc in skin healing processes
- Ceramides —build the lipid barrier

At the stage of planning the peeling procedure, for subsequent monitoring of skin recovery, and in the evaluation of the clinical results achieved and their duration, instrumental methods of skin condition analysis can be successfully applied. We will focus on them next.

More information about skincare products for rehabilitation is available in the *Comprehensive Cosmetic Skincare in Cosmetic Dermatology & Skincare Practice* book.

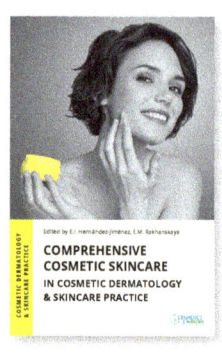

Part IV

Instrumental assessment of skin condition and after-peeling support of barrier function

Regardless of the clinical result, chemical peeling is additional stress and, even if controlled, causes damage to the skin. The professional peel procedure should be accompanied by monitoring of the skin functional characteristics using instrumental methods to ensure maximal safety and efficacy (Berardesca E. et al., 2014; Antonov D. et al., 2016). The information obtained helps us understand how the skin reacts to chemical peels and provides objective criteria for the construction of a post-procedural skin care program (Trojahn C. et al., 2015; Giménez-Arnau A., 2016; Döge N. et al., 2017).

1.1. Symptoms of skin damage after chemical peeling

Regardless of the goal — whether it is to rejuvenate the skin, remove pigmentation, or correct hyperkeratosis — the effect of any chemical peeling is based on the damage and subsequent regeneration of the skin (Song J.Y. et al., 2004).

The required depth of damage is "set" by choosing the type of peel, the concentration of the peeling agent in it, pH (in acid peel), and exposure time (Rubio L. et al., 2011). With the competent use of chemical peel, the induced damage is usually enough to activate the skin's natural reparative processes and achieve the desired effect without any complications.

Peels are almost always accompanied by two undesirable reactions — erythema and visible scaling. Erythema is one of the main clinical symptoms that the skincare specialist should focus on to assess the safety and depth of skin damage. After superficial peel, redness lasting up to a day is considered normal, although usually, after glycolic peeling, erythema lasts from 20 minutes to two hours. With superficial and medium-depth peel, the erythema may last up to two days, with medium-depth TCA peeling up to a week, and in some cases for 2–3 weeks.

Transient erythema is not an inflammation but a skin reaction to chemical irritation. The mechanism of redness is related to the irritation of nociceptive receptors of slow C-afferent fibers located in the epidermis. Blocking these receptors (e.g., with strontium nitrate) significantly reduces the irritation caused by glycolic acid. The prolonged persistent erythema is evidence of damage and inflammation in the deeper layers of the skin. Multiple pinpoint hemorrhages, and effusion of tissue fluid with subsequent formation of a scab, which disappears on its own within two weeks, are noted. The duration of subsequent erythema and inflammatory reaction in deep peels can last several months.

The second obligatory effect of the peel, which is relatively easy to determine clinically, is visible scaling. Its nature depends on the peel type. In the case of superficial acid peel, slight scaling appears on Day 2–3 after the procedure. In the case of keratolytic peel, during the procedure, denatured protein mass begins to depart in the form of a frost, and a few days later a true exfoliation of horny scales in the form of light powdering may be observed. After enzymatic peels, exfoliation is usually not visible. Retinol peel, on the other hand, leads to desquamation a few days after the treatment.

As a result of damage to the barrier properties, the ability of the *stratum corneum* to regulate and maintain the necessary water level is temporarily lost, causing a decline in hydration. Therefore, in addition to the visible symptoms of damage in the form of erythema and scaling, almost any peel causes subjective symptoms of dry skin — a feeling of tightness, sometimes itching and burning (**Fig. IV-1-1**).

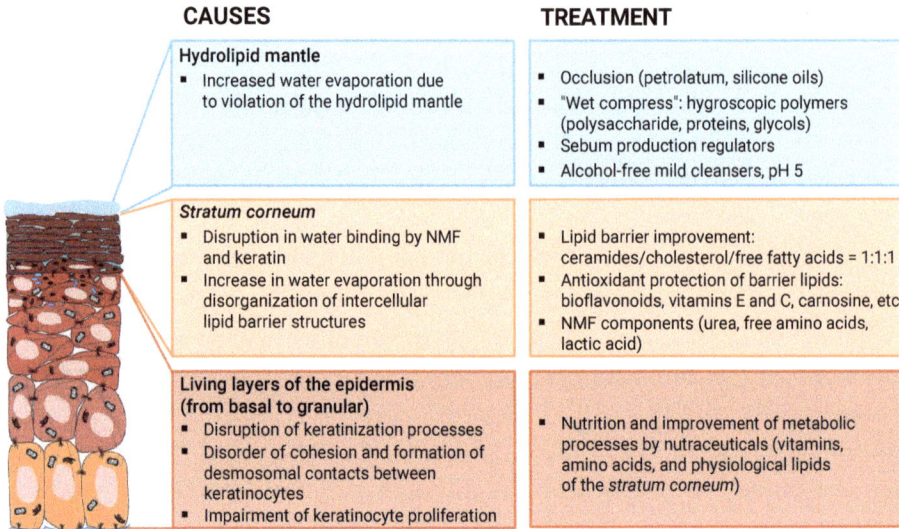

Figure IV-1-1. Dry skin: causes and ways to treat it

1.2. Post-peeling dryness: causes, assessment, treatment

The main mechanisms of disruption of the water balance in the epidermis include:
1. Intercellular contacts disorder and desquamation alteration
2. Disorganization of intercellular lipid matrix
3. Changes in the sebum production
4. Disruption of water binding and retention in the epidermis

For each of these mechanisms, methods have been developed to assess the degree of their impairment. A comprehensive measurement of the various functional characteristics allows an accurate assessment of the skin condition already in the early stages of water imbalance and a targeted effect on the main pathophysiological mechanisms that lead to dry skin (**Fig. IV-1-1**). The most important methods that are used to evaluate dry skin and the results of the peeling are shown in **Fig. IV-1-2** and **IV-1-3** and **Table IV-1-1**.

Sebumetry: skin oiliness assessment

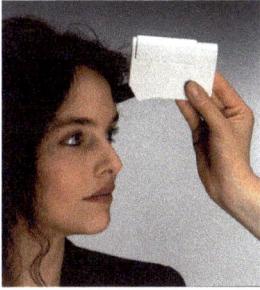

The measurement is based on grease spot photometry. The matte tape of the Sebumeter® SM 815 is brought into contact with skin or hair. It becomes transparent according to the sebum on the surface of the measurement area. Then the tape is inserted into the aperture of the device and its transparency is measured by a photocell. The light transmission represents the sebum content.

Corneometry: quantitative determination of the *stratum corneum* hydration degree

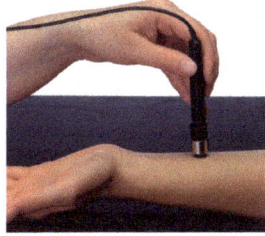

It is based on capacitance measurement of a dielectric constant of the *stratum corneum* at a depth of 0.1 mm. The dielectric constant will change with water content

Tewametry: quantitative transepidermal water loss determination

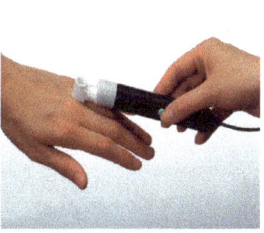

The Tewameter® probe measures the density gradient of the water evaporation from the skin indirectly by the two pairs of sensors (temperature and relative humidity) inside the hollow cylinder. This is an "open chamber" measurement method

Figure IV-1-2. Skin analysis methods that can be used to determine the degree and causes of dryness (CK electronic GmbH, Germany)

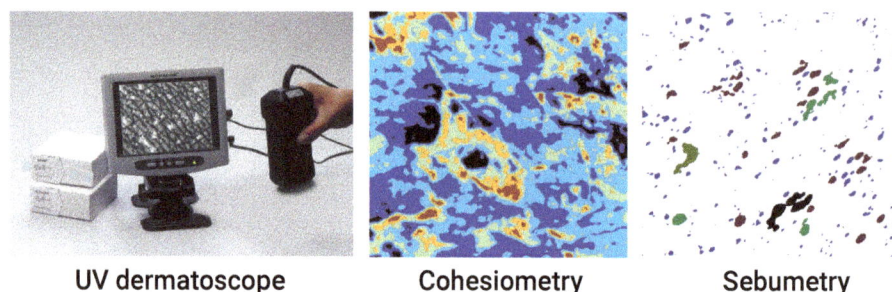

| UV dermatoscope | Cohesiometry | Sebumetry |

Figure IV-1-3. Imaging techniques (CK electronic GmbH, Germany)

UV dermatoscope is used to analyze the appearance of a special film.

Cohesiometry: corneocytes adhere to the adhesive film — the thicker they are, the lighter they are in ultraviolet light (the figure shows a cohesiogram after treatment, the lighter and thicker corneocytes are highlighted in red).

Sebumetry: after the film is applied to the skin, it changes its transparency — the more active the sebaceous gland is, the larger the spot it leaves on the film (the figure shows a sebogram after computer processing, sebaceous spots of different sizes are highlighted in color).

Table IV-1-1. Basic methods for evaluating the clinical results of peeling

METHOD	EVALUATION PARAMETER
Cohesiometry	• Degree of scaling and strength of adhesion between corneocytes
Tewametry	• Disruption of barrier properties and organization of intercellular lipid matrix
Sebumetry	• Sebostatic effect: effect on sebum production and formation of an oily film on the skin surface
Corneometry	• Dry skin: binding and retaining water in the *stratum corneum*
UV visualization	• Microrelief • Desquamation
Mexametry	• Erythema: microcirculation, irritation, inflammation • Pigmentation: whitening effect • Complications in the form of hyper- and hypopigmentation

1.2.1. Desquamation

Visible scaling is one of the criteria for the effectiveness of chemical peels in renewing the epidermal cell composition. The severity and nature of this symptom vary depending on the peeling agent's chemical nature and concentration and exposure time. Epidermal cells are bound together with desmosomes that maintain the integrity of the tissue itself and limit the diffusion of substances (including water) into the intercellular space. The tighter the cells adhere to each other, the harder it is for water and dissolved substances to seep between them.

As keratinocytes move to the epidermis surface, the number of intercellular desmosomal contacts increases, and the width of intercellular gaps decreases. The *stratum corneum* is the most compact — in it, corneocytes adhere tightly to each other and are interconnected by a large number of corneodesmosomes. The chemical peeling agent destroys not only the existing corneodesmosomes, but also inhibits their formation. This results in the weakening of the intercellular bonds, and the corneocytes leave the skin surface more quickly — this process is called desquamation.

Cohesiometry is used to objectively assess the degree of scaling (Riethmüller C., 2018). For this purpose, special films are utilized on which corneocytes adhere in contact with the skin. The number, size, and shape of these scales are used to judge the nature of *stratum corneum* desquamation. Special UV dermatoscopes (visioscopes) — and in some cases microscopes — are used to obtain images (**Fig. IV-1-4**).

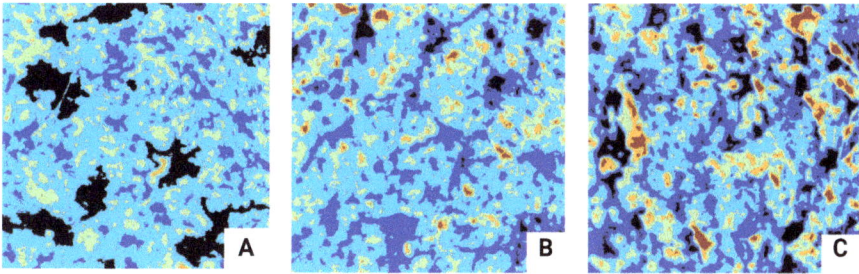

Figure IV-1-4. Cohesiogram: A — physiological desquamation (normal); B — uniform desquamation of small corneocytes after superficial acid peeling; C — large scales after medium-depth TCA peeling. Color corresponds to the thickness of corneocytes — from thin (dark blue) to thick (red), black — no scaling (CK electronic GmbH, Germany)

Normally, a certain number of thin corneocytes constantly slough off the skin surface. An increase in their surface area and thickness can be seen on a cohesiogram already in the early stages of desquamation disorders when there are no visible signs of scaling yet. Enzymatic and mild acid peels usually cause a uniform exfoliation of small corneocytes that may be barely visible or invisible. After a stronger acid peel, the scaling becomes noticeable, but it is still different from the coarse scales resulting from a retinol peel or a medium-depth TCA peeling. When the living layers of the epidermis are exposed, the keratinization process is affected at an earlier stage, resulting in the formation of corneocytes that differ in appearance and strength of adhesion to each other.

1.2.2. Transepidermal water loss

After even superficial peels, there is a significant increase in transepidermal water loss (TEWL). This is a result of the chemical agent's action:
- The *stratum corneum* is loosened and/or partially removed.
- The corneodesmosomal connections between the corneocytes are damaged.
- The integrity of the intercellular lipid matrix is disrupted.

The lipid barrier (lipid layer filling the space between corneocytes) starts to form at the border of the epidermis's granular layer and the *stratum corneum*. Intercellular contacts providing mechanical integrity of the epidermis are an essential element of the skin barrier. After superficial peel, the barrier is restored relatively quickly. However, the granular layer is damaged in the case of medium-depth peel. Therefore, the barrier function restoration requires a much longer period and a more intensive course of post-peel care.

Lipid matrix plays an important role in the regulation of water balance, and its disruption is a frequent cause of skin dryness, but this fact sometimes escapes the attention of skincare specialists. The reason is that the lipid matrix is hidden from the eye and can only be assessed by instrumental means, using the method of tewametry, which measures the rate of water evaporation from the skin surface (see **Fig. IV-1-2**). The TEWL index depends not only on the state of the intercellular matrix and corneodesmosomal contacts but also on several other parameters. In particular, it is influenced by the activity of sweat and sebaceous glands, so cleaning the skin prior to the measurements ensures that these factors do not impact the findings.

Unsaturated fatty acids in the lipids of the intercellular matrix are an excellent target for oxidizing agents and UV rays, which trigger lipid peroxidation in the intercellular lipid barrier. This disturbs the intercellular matrix's structural organization, leading to an increase in TEWL and dehydration of the *stratum corneum*. This should be kept in mind during post-peel care, especially in the summer.

It is advisable not only to prescribe cosmetics to restore the lipid intercellular layer but also to protect it from free-radical oxidation. Most often, antioxidants — vitamin E, bioflavonoids, and histidine-containing dipeptides (carnosine, anserine) — are used for this purpose, interrupting the ipid peroxidation chain reaction. A combination of lipids comprising the lipid barrier — ceramides, cholesterol, and free fatty acids in a 1:1:1 ratio — can theoretically be used to restore the lipid barrier. It has been shown that this ratio of components provides the most effective restoration of the skin barrier function. But in practice, such mixtures are not used for such purposes due to the high cost of ceramides, the presence of which in the composition of restorative preparations is highly desirable.

For a rapid reduction of TEWL, it is advisable and justified to use occlusive agents. Targeted treatment and restoration of the intercellular lipid matrix is carried out not only by cosmetic means but also by nutritional correction and intake of nutraceuticals containing ceramides and unsaturated fatty acids to restore the skin lipid matrix "from within" (Zhang Z. et al., 2018). As a preventive measure, sunscreens should be used, as their application can significantly reduce the processes of peroxidation in the summer.

1.2.3. Sebum

The importance of sebum in the pathogenesis of dry skin cannot be underestimated — degreasing the skin with an alcohol solution removes the hydrolipid mantle, and, as a consequence, the TEWL and skin permeability to water-soluble substances immediately increase.

One of the peel procedure stages is skin cleansing (including sebum) which, in addition to the aggressive action of peeling agents, further reduces the skin's barrier function. Therefore, after completing any peel procedure and in the early post-peel period, special attention should be paid to the occlusion of the skin. To do this, creating an artificial layer on its surface is necessary to imitate the hydrolipid mantle. As a rule, waxes, high-molecular-weight silicone oils, mineral oil, and Vaseline give a good occlusion effect.

Care is needed with some hygroscopic polymers (e.g., hyaluronic acid, propylene glycols), even though they are widely used to moisturize the skin. The fact is that, after application, they remain on the skin surface, and the water with which they are impregnated quickly evaporates. Therefore, gel serums are not the products of choice for skin with a compromised barrier.

It should be understood that water flows from the inside out, and the TEWL index is always positive. By creating a thin film of hygroscopic polymers on the skin surface, we provide only emergency hydration, which is relatively short-lived. After the water contained in such a surface coating has completely evaporated, the dried hygroscopic polymers begin to dry out and cling to the skin surface, tightening the skin. Therefore, without additional occlusion, the patient soon begins to feel discomfort and symptoms of dry skin. This is especially noticeable in dry and windy climates. Because of this feature, **gels and serums can be considered only as additional means of emergency moisturizing, over which it is necessary to apply emulsion preparation with occlusive ingredients — only in this case it is possible to moisturize the skin for a long time**.

Before prescribing post-peel care products, it is necessary to understand the mechanism of their action. The first guideline is the ingredient composition of the cosmetic product. However, before prescribing, it is advisable to test all available products from the cosmetic line to understand how they behave when used. For this purpose, it is necessary to measure moisturization and TEWL index of the patient's skin before the application of the preparation (initial value) and 15–20 minutes after the application. The criterion for the effectiveness of the occlusion is a decrease in TEWL and an increase in skin hydration compared to the initial values (**Fig. IV-1-5**).

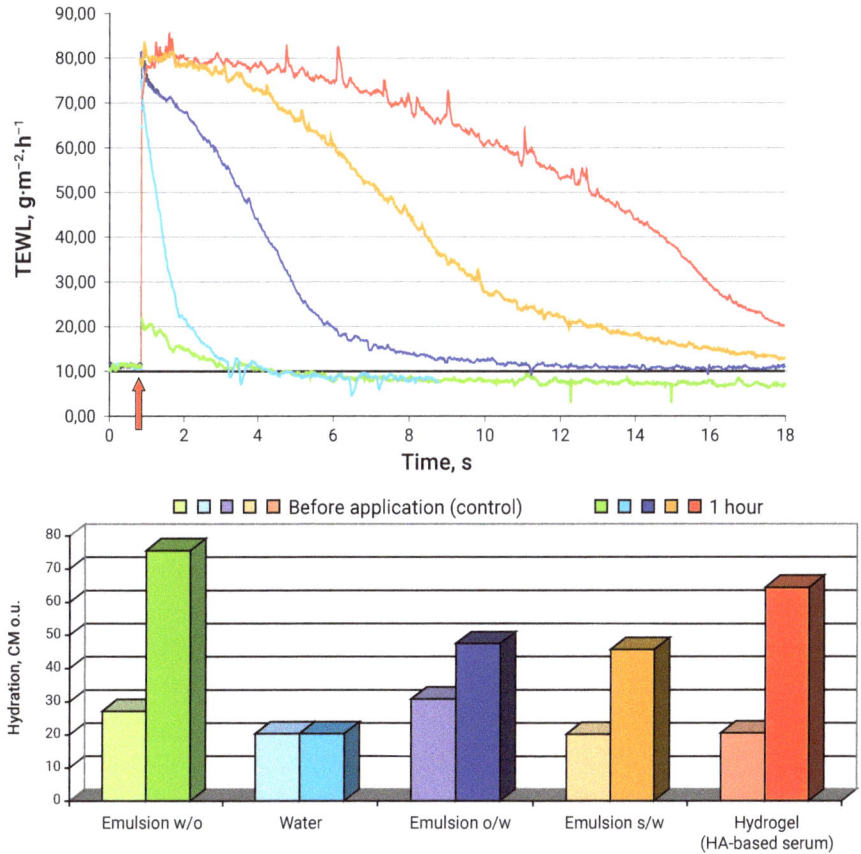

Figure IV-1-5. Changes in (A) TEWL and (B) hydration as a result of topically applied preparations with different water content and different bases

When a cosmetic product containing water is applied to the skin, there is an increase in the evaporation of water from the surface (this can be observed using tewametry — the TEWL index increases). The dynamics of water evaporation depend on the product type and the amount of water it contains.

- The **water-in-oil emulsion (w/o)** contains relatively few water droplets suspended in the oil phase. After it is applied to the skin, the TEWL index increases; after three minutes only, it returns to the initial state. After seven minutes, it becomes lower than the initial value, which indicates occlusion due to the components of the oil phase.
- **Oil-in-water (o/w)** and **silicone-in-water (s/w)** emulsions have similar TEWL index dynamics. Since they contain more water than the water-in-oil emulsions, the increased TEWL index persists for a longer time, and the moisturizing effect is less pronounced.
- Once the **hydrogel** is applied to the skin, water evaporates from it intensively, reflecting the high TEWL index. The rate of evaporation depends on climatic conditions — the drier the air, the faster the evaporation. Evaporation rate is also affected by temperature and wind. However, due to the water-holding capacity of hyaluronic acid, water evaporates much slower than when skin is moisturized with just water.

Note that, when sebaceous glands become more active, the quantity and the quality of the sebum secreted by them often change. Sebum becomes more liquid and seeps through the intercellular spaces, gradually changing the composition and structure of intercellular lipid layers. The disorganized lipid barrier is less able to retain water flow, resulting in an increase in the TEWL index and decreased hydration of the *stratum corneum*.

It is no coincidence that seborrheic skin is dry! In this case, a course of superficial salicylic peel treatments can be performed to normalize the sebaceous glands, which eventually affects the restoration of the barrier properties of the *stratum corneum*. The correct post-peel care consolidates the results achieved.

As a rule, assessing impaired sebum production and associated dry skin is not difficult. Depending on the activity of sebum secretion, the following skin types are distinguished:

- Normal skin — with normal sebum production
- Low-sebum skin — with insufficient sebum production
- Oily skin — with increased sebum discharge

The skin type can be easily determined by external examination of the patient based on clinical signs. Nevertheless, in practice, there is a need for objective evaluation criteria, both to clarify the skin condition and to monitor the effectiveness of skincare interventions, such as sebostatic agents or cleansing procedures. Sebumetry is recognized as the reference method for skin evaluation. It works on the principle that, in contact with the skin, a special matte film absorbs sebum and becomes more transparent. For quantification, either a photometric measurement of the absolute amount of sebum (in ng/cm^2) is made (see **Fig. IV-1-2**), or the film is photographed in advance with a dermatoscope (visioscope) for subsequent analysis of the number and size of sebum spots (see **Fig. IV-1-3**).

1.2.4. Hydration

When we talk about cosmetic skin hydration, we refer to hydration of the *stratum corneum* — if the moisture level in the *stratum corneum* is below normal. Extra hydration can lead to hyper-hydration, which is not beneficial if hydration is normal. It is still important to make sure your skin is properly hydrated before using moisturizers.

An instrumental method for assessing moisture levels is corneometry, based on the measurement of the dielectric constant (see **Fig. IV-1-2**). With this method, the hydration of only the "dead" *stratum corneum*, in which there is little water (on average 15% by weight), but it is still present, is assessed. Measurement of hydration of deeper "living" layers of epidermis and even more so of derma is inexpedient, since water content in them reaches 80% and more — aqueous environment is necessary to ensure normal vital activity of cells.

It is in the *stratum corneum* and on its surface that subtle mechanisms of water balance regulation operate. Besides the intercellular (lipid barrier) and superficial (sebum) lipids discussed above, there are two more very important water-holding structures that bind water:
- Keratin — a high-molecular-weight protein inside the corneocytes
- Natural moisturizing factor — small hygroscopic molecules (free amino acids, urea, lactic acid, sodium pyroglutamate) around the corneocytes

Water is bound to these substances by ionic bonds. The post-peel dryness of the skin is partly caused by the decrease in the content of these substances in the *stratum corneum*. The inclusion of natural moisturizing factor components in post-peel products is thus advisable. Nanoemulsion-based formulations are suitable for deeper delivery of moisturizing ingredients. With the help of corneometry, it is possible to monitor the restoration rate of the water-retaining structures in the *stratum corneum* (Stettler H. et al., 2017; Angelova-Fischer I. et al., 2018).

1.3. Comprehensive approach to the assessment and treatment of dryness

The peel procedure is a serious damaging factor leading to dry and flaky skin. In patients with pre-existing symptoms of dry skin, it is important to assess the following functional characteristics of the skin at the initial consultation:

1. Hydration
2. TEWL index
3. Sebum production
4. Scaling intensity

Only a comprehensive assessment of these parameters allows you to identify the leading causes of dry skin and prescribe optimal skin preparation for the subsequent scaling. Prolonged application of peeling agents damages the skin even more. Periodic monitoring of objective indicators is desirable to allow time to adjust skincare between treatments and to select supportive care after the course.

The frequency of measurements is determined individually. For example, if the prescribed remedy or procedure aims to eliminate dry skin symptoms rapidly, the effect should be evaluated after the procedure or application of cosmetics. If the efforts are aimed not at the symptomatic elimination of dryness but at the normalization of the lipid barrier, the persistent moisturizing effect manifests itself only after the entire course of care. In this case, it is advisable to evaluate the effectiveness in the middle and at the end of the course of treatment.

Chemical peeling is often described as "controlled skin damage," implying that the skincare practitioner monitors the degree of damage and does not allow the skin to cross the line beyond which the risks are too high. The skin is damaged to initiate recovery processes, which must also be monitored. Previously, experts used to control all stages of the peeling "by eye," but now they have the tools of objective control, which considerably reduces the likelihood of complications and increases the treatment effectiveness.

References

Ajlia S.A., Majid F.A., Suvik A. et al. Efficacy of papain-based wound cleanser in promoting wound regeneration. Pak J Biol Sci 2010; 13(12): 596–603.

Angelova-Fischer I., Fischer T.W., Abels C. et al. Accelerated barrier recovery and enhancement of the barrier integrity and properties by topical application of a pH 4 vs a pH 5.8 water-in-oil emulsion in aged skin. Br J Dermatol 2018; 179(2): 471–477.

Antonov D., Schliemann S., Elsner P. Methods for the assessment of barrier function. Curr Probl Dermatol 2016; 49: 61–70.

Aubert J., Piwnica D., Bertino B. et al. Nonclinical and human pharmacology of the potent and selective topical retinoic acid receptor-γ agonist trifarotene. Br J Dermatol 2018; 179(2): 442–456.

Balak D.M.W. Topical trifarotene: a new retinoid. Br J Dermatol 2018; 179(2): 231–232.

Berardesca E., Distante F., Vignoli G.P. et al. Alpha hydroxyacids modulate stratum corneum barrier function. Br J Dermatol 1997; 137(6): 934–938.

Berardesca E., Maibach H.I., Wilhelm K.-P. (eds.). Non-invasive diagnostic techniques in clinical dermatology. Springer, 2014.

Blomhoff R., Blomhoff H.K. Overview of retinoid metabolism and function. J Neurobiol 2006; 66(7): 606–630.

Brocklehurst K., Philpott M.P. Cysteine proteases: mode of action and role in epidermal differentiation. Cell Tissue Res 2013; 351(2): 237–244. Review.

Brody H.J. Segmental chemical peeling medium and deep peels. Presented at 5CC, August 31, 2018.

Brody H.J., Hailey C.W. Medium-depth peeling of the skin: a variation of superficial chemo-surgery. J Dermatol Surg Oncl 1986; 12: 1268–1275.

Buslaeva E.R. PQAge (Promoitalia): an innovative technology for chemical skin remodeling. Cosmetics and Medicine 2016; 4: 88–93.

Caubet C., Jonca N., Brattsand M. et al. Degradation of corneodesmosome proteins by two serine proteases of the kallikrein family, SCTE/KLK5/hK5 and SCCE/KLK7/hK7. J Invest Dermatol 2004; 122(5): 1235–1244.

Chaudhuri R.K., Bojanowski K. Bakuchiol: a retinol-like functional compound revealed by gene expression profiling and clinically proven to have anti-aging effects. Int J Cosmet Sci 2014; 36(3): 221–230.

Choi E.H., Man M.Q., Xu P. et al. Stratum corneum acidification is impaired in moderately aged human and murine skin. J Invest Dermatol 2007; 127(12): 2847–2856.

Choi J.E., Di Nardo A. Skin neurogenic inflammation. Seminars Immunopathol 2018; 40(3): 249–259.

Coleman D.J., Garcia G., Hyter S. et al. Retinoid-X-receptors (α/β) in melanocytes modulate innate immune responses and differentially regulate cell survival following UV irradiation. PLoS Genet 2014; 10(5): e1004321.

Coleman W.P., Futrell J.M. The glycolic acid + trichloracetic acid peel. J Dermatol Surg Oncol 1994; 20(1): 76–80.

Cork M.J, Danby S.G., Vasilopoulos Y. et al. Epidermal barrier dysfunction in atopic dermatitis. J Invest Dermatol 2009; 129(8): 1892–1908.

Descargues P., Deraison C., Prost C. et al. Corneodesmosomal cadherins are preferential targets of stratum corneum trypsin- and chymotrypsin-like hyperactivity in Netherton syndrome. J Invest Dermatol 2006; 126(7): 1622–1632.

Dhaliwal S., Rybak I., Ellis S.R. et al. Prospective, randomized, double-blind assessment of topical bakuchiol and retinol for facial photoaging. Br J Dermatol 2019; 180(2): 289–296.

Döge N., Avetisyan A., Hadam S. et al. Assessment of skin barrier function and biochemical changes of ex vivo human skin in response to physical and chemical barrier disruption. Eur J Pharm Biopharm 2017; 116: 138–148.

Downs J.W., Wills B.K. Phenol toxicity. StatPearls Publishing, 2020.

Egberts F., Heinrich M., Jensen J.-M. et al. Cathepsin D is involved in the regulation of transglutaminase 1 and epidermal differentiation. J Cell Sci 2004;117(Pt 11): 2295–2307.

Elias P.M., Wakefield J.S. Mechanisms of abnormal lamellar body secretion and the dysfunctional skin barrier in patients with atopic dermatitis. J Allergy Clin Immunol 2014; 134(4): 781–791.

Evans R.M., Mangelsdorf D.J. Nuclear receptors, RXR, and the Big Bang. Cell 2014; 157(1): 255–266.

Fisher C., Blumenberg M., Tomić-Canić M. Retinoid receptors and keratinocytes. Crit Rev Oral Biol Med 1995; 6(4): 284–301.

Fortugno P., Furio L., Teson M. et al. The 420K LEKTI variant alters LEKTI proteolytic activation and results in protease deregulation: implications for atopic dermatitis. Hum Mol Genet 2012; 21(19): 4187–4200.

Fuchs K.O., Solis O., Tapawan R., Paranjpe J. The effects of an estrogen and glycolic acid cream on the facial skin of postmenopausal women: a randomized histologic study. Cutis 2003; 71(6): 481–488.

Galliano M.F., Toulza E., Gallinaro H. et al. A novel protease inhibitor of the alpha2-macroglobulin family expressed in the human epidermis. J Biol Chem 2006; 281(9): 5780–5789.

Giménez-Arnau A. Standards for the protection of skin barrier function. Curr Probl Dermatol 2016; 49: 123–134.

Grimes P.E. Jessner's solution. In: Tosti A., Grimes P.E., De Padova M.P. (eds.), Color Atlas of Chemical Peels. Springer, 2006; pp. 23–29.

Hanson K.M., Behne M.J., Barry N.P. et al. Two-photon fluorescence lifetime imaging of the skin stratum corneum pH gradient. Biophys J 2002; 83(3): 1682–1590.

Has C. Peeling skin disorders: a paradigm for skin desquamation. J Invest Dermatol 2018; 138(8): 1689–1691.

Hetter G.P. An examination of the phenol-croton oil peel: Part I. Dissecting the formula. Plast Reconstr Surg 2000a; 105(1): 227–239; discussion 249–251.

Hetter G.P. An examination of the phenol-croton oil peel: Part II. The lay peelers and their croton oil formulas. Plast Reconstr Surg 2000b;105(1): 240–248; discussion 249–251.

Hetter G.P. An examination of the phenol-croton oil peel: Part III. The plastic surgeons' role. Plast Reconstr Surg 2000c; 105(2): 752–763.

Hetter G.P. An examination of the phenol-croton oil peel: Part IV. Face peel results with different concentrations of phenol and croton oil. Plast Reconstr Surg 2000d; 105(3): 1061–1083; discussion 1084–1087.

Horikoshi T., Igarashi S., Uchiwa H. et al. Role of endogenous cathepsin D-like and chymotrypsin-like proteolysis in human epidermal desquamation. Br J Dermatol 1999; 141(3): 453–459.

Howell J.B., Beck T., Bates B. et al. Interaction of alpha 2-macroglobulin with trypsin, chymotrypsin, plasmin, and papain. Arch Biochem Biophys 1983; 221(1): 261–270.

Huang N., Mi T., Xu S. et al. Traffic-derived air pollution compromises skin barrier function and stratum corneum redox status: a population study. J Cosmet Dermatol 2020; 19(7): 1751–1759.

Hung S.J., Tang S.C., Liao P.Y. et al. Photoprotective potential of glycolic acid by reducing NLRC4 and AIM2 inflammasome complex proteins in UVB radiation-induced normal human epidermal keratinocytes and mice. DNA Cell Biol 2017; 36(2): 177–187.

Igarashi S., Takizawa T., Takizawa T. et al. Cathepsin D, but not cathepsin E, degrades desmosomes during epidermal desquamation. Br J Dermatol 2004; 151(2): 355–361.

Ishida-Yamamoto A., Igawa S., Kishibe M. Order and disorder in corneocyte adhesion. J Dermatol 2011; 38(7): 645–654.

Iuchi K., Morisada Y., Yoshino Y. et al. Cold atmospheric-pressure nitrogen plasma induces the production of reactive nitrogen species and cell death by increasing intracellular calcium in HEK293T cells. Arch Biochem Biophys 2018; 654: 136–145.

Jaffary F., Faghihi G., Saraeian S., Hosseini S.M. Comparison the effectiveness of pyruvic acid 50% and salicylic acid 30% in the treatment of acne. J Res Med Sci 2016; 21: 31.

Johnson J.B., Ichinose H., Obagi Z.E., Laub D.R. Obagi's modified trichloroacetic acid (TCA)-controlled variable-depth peel: a study of clinical signs correlating with histological findings. Ann Plast Surg 1996; 36(3): 225–237.

Justo A.D.S., Lemes B.M., Nunes B. et al. Depth of injury of Hetter's phenol–croton oil chemical peel formula using 2 different emulsifying agents. J Am Acad Dermatol 2020; 82(6): 1544–1546.

Kang S. The mechanism of action of topical retinoids. Cutis 2005; 75(2 Suppl): 10–13.

Karlsson C., Andersson M.L., Collin M. et al. SufA — a novel subtilisin-like serine proteinase of Finegoldia magna. Microbiology 2007; 153(Pt 12): 4208–4218.

Khalil S., Bardawil T., Stephan C. et al. Retinoids: a journey from the molecular structures and mechanisms of action to clinical uses in dermatology and adverse effects. J Dermatolog Treat 2017; 28(8): 684–696.

Kim M.J., Ciletti N., Michel S. et al. The role of specific retinoid receptors in sebocyte growth and differentiation in culture. J Invest Dermatol 2000; 114(2): 349–253.

Komatsu N., Saijoh K., Kuk C. et al. Aberrant human tissue kallikrein levels in the stratum corneum and serum of patients with psoriasis: dependence on phenotype, severity and therapy. Br J Dermatol 2007; 156(5): 875–883.

Korneeva R.V., Voytenko I.V. Armorique IO PRC: technology of noninvasive skin remodeling and rejuvenation using a new generation of modified trichloroacetic acid-based products. Cosmetics and Medicine 2019; 1: 27–34.

Krężel W., Rühl R., de Lera A.R. Alternative retinoid X receptor (RXR) ligands. Mol Cell Endocrinol 2019; 491: 110436.

Larange A., Cheroutre H. Retinoic acid and retinoic acid receptors as pleiotropic modulators of the immune system. Annu Rev Immunol 2016; 34: 369–394.

Larson D.L., Karmo F., Hetter G.P. Phenol–croton oil peel: establishing an animal model for scientific investigation. Aesthet Surg J 2009; 29(1): 47–53.

Lee A.-Y. Molecular mechanism of epidermal barrier dysfunction as primary abnormalities. Int J Mol Sci 2020; 21(4): 1194.

Lee B., Heo J., Hong S., Kim E.Y. et al. DL-malic acid as a component of α-hydroxy acids: effect on 2,4-dinitrochlorobenzene-induced inflammation in atopic dermatitis-like skin lesions in vitro and in vivo. Immunopharmacol Immunotoxicol 2019; 41(6): 614–621.

Lee J.B., Chung W.G., Kwahck H., Lee K.H. Focal treatment of acne scars with trichloroacetic acid: chemical reconstruction of skin scars method. Dermatol Surg 2002; 28(11): 1017–1021.

Lee J.C., Daniels M.A., Roth M.Z. Mesotherapy, microneedling, and chemical peels. Clin Plast Surg 2016; 43(3): 583–595.

Lee K.C., Wambier C.G., Soon S.L. et al. Basic chemical peeling: superficial and medium-depth peels. J Am Acad Dermatol 2019; 81(2): 313–324.

Li J., Li Q., Geng S. All-trans-retinoic acid alters the expression of the tight junction proteins Claudin 1 and 4 and epidermal barrier function-associated genes in the epidermis. Int J Mol Med 2019; 43(4): 1789–1805.

Lu J., Cong T., Wen X. et al. Salicylic acid treats acne vulgaris by suppressing AMPK/SREBP1 pathway in sebocytes. Exp Dermatol 2019; 28(7): 786–794.

Lu Z., Xie Y., Huang H. et al. Hair follicle stem cells regulate retinoid metabolism to maintain the self-renewal niche for melanocyte stem cells. Elife. 2020; 9: e52712.

Matsubara Y., Matsumoto T., Koseki J. et al. Inhibition of human kallikrein 5 protease by triterpenoids from natural sources. Molecules 2017; 22(11): 1829.

Maurer H.R. Bromelain: biochemistry, pharmacology and medical use. Cell Mol Life Sci 2001; 58(9): 1234–1245.

Meunier L., Bohjanen K., Voorhees J.J. et al. Retinoic acid upregulates human Langerhans cell antigen presentation and surface expression of HLA-DR and CD11c, a beta 2 integrin critically involved in T-cell activation. J Invest Dermatol 1994; 103(6): 775–779.

Meyer-Hoffert U. Reddish, scaly, and itchy: how proteases and their inhibitors contribute to inflammatory skin diseases. Arch Immunol Ther Exp (Warsz) 2009; 57(5): 345–354.

Monheit G.D. The Jessner's + TCA peel: a medium-depth chemical peel. Dermatol Surg 1989; 15: 945–950.

Napoli J.L. Cellular retinoid binding-proteins, CRBP, CRABP, FABP5: effects on retinoid metabolism, function and related diseases. Pharmacol Ther 2017; 173: 19–33.

Nylander-Lundqvist E., Egelrud T. Formation of active IL-1 beta from pro-IL-1 beta catalyzed by stratum corneum chymotryptic enzyme in vitro. Acta Derm Venereol 1997; 77(3): 203–206.

Obagi Z.E., Obagi S., Alaiti S. et al. TCA-based blue peel: a standardized procedure with depth control. Dermatol Surg 1999; 25(10): 773–780.

O'Connor A.A., Lowe P.M., Shumack S. et al. Chemical peels: a review of current practice. Australas J Dermatol 2018; 59(3): 171–181.

Oliveira L.M., Teixeira F.M.E., Sato M.N. Impact of retinoic acid on immune cells and inflammatory diseases. Mediators Inflamm 2018; 2018: 3067126.

Palmieri B., Vadala M., Laurino C. Nutrition in wound healing: investigation of the molecular mechanisms, a narrative review. J Wound Care 2019; 28(10): 683–691.

Pawar N.R., Buzza M.S., Antalis T.M. Membrane-anchored serine proteases and protease-activated receptor-2-mediated signaling: co-conspirators in cancer progression. Cancer Res 2019; 79(2): 301–310.

Petkovich M., Brand N.J., Krust A., Chambon P. A human retinoic acid receptor which belongs to the family of nuclear receptors. Nature 1987; 330(6147): 444–450.

Rawlings A.V., Voegeli R. Stratum corneum proteases and dry skin conditions. Cell Tissue Res 2013; 351(2): 217–235.

Reddy V.B., Lerner E.A. Plant cysteine proteases that evoke itch activate protease-activated receptors. Br J Dermatol 2010; 163(3): 532–535.

Riahi R.R., Bush A.E., Cohen P.R. Topical retinoids: therapeutic mechanisms in the treatment of photodamaged skin. Am J Clin Dermatol 2016; 17(3): 265–276.

Riethmüller C. Assessing the skin barrier via corneocyte morphometry. Exp Dermatol 2018; 27(8): 923–930.

Rubio L., Alonso C., López O. et al. Barrier function of intact and impaired skin: percutaneous penetration of caffeine and salicylic acid. Int J Dermatol 2011; 50(7): 881–889.

Saldanha S., Royston K., Udayakumar N., Tollefsbol T. Epigenetic regulation of epidermal stem cell biomarkers and their role in wound healing. Int J Mol Sci 2015; 17(1): 16.

Scott L.J. Trifarotene: first approval. Drugs 2019; 79(17): 1905–1909.

Shai A.M. DSA peels and REPART® biorevitalizants are an effective comprehensive approach to skin rejuvenation. Injection Methods in Cosmetology 2019; 4: 100–105.

Shao Y., He T., Fisher G.J. et al. Molecular basis of retinol anti-ageing properties in naturally aged human skin in vivo. Int J Cosmet Sci 2017; 39(1): 56–65.

Sharma A., Goren A., Dhurat R. et al. Tretinoin enhances minoxidil response in androgenetic alopecia patients by upregulating follicular sulfotransferase enzymes. Dermatol Ther 2019; 32(3): 12915.

Song J.Y., Kang H.A., Kim M.Y. et al. Damage and recovery of skin barrier function after glycolic acid chemical peeling and crystal microdermabrasion. Dermatol Surg 2004; 30(3): 390–394.

Stahl W., Sies H. β-Carotene and other carotenoids in protection from sunlight. Am J Clin Nutr 2012; 96(5): 1179–1184.

Starkman S.J., Mangat D.S. Chemical peel (deep, medium, light). Facial Plast Surg Clin North Am 2020; 28(1): 45–57.

Stettler H., Kurka P., Lunau N. et al. A new topical panthenol-containing emollient: results from two randomized controlled studies assessing its skin moisturization and barrier restoration potential, and the effect on skin microflora. J Dermatolog Treat 2017; 28(2): 173–180.

Sun H.F., Lu H.S., Sun L.Q. et al. Chemical peeling with a modified phenol formula for the treatment of facial freckles on Asian skin. Aesthetic Plast Surg 2018; 42(2): 546–552.

Tang S.-C., Tang L.-C., Liu C.-H. et al. Glycolic acid attenuates UVB-induced aquaporin-3, matrix metalloproteinase-9 expression, and collagen degradation in keratinocytes and mouse skin. Biochem J 2019; 476(10): 1387–1400.

Tang S.-C., Yang J.-H. Dual effects of alpha-hydroxy acids on the skin. Molecules 2018; 23: 863.

Tasić-Kostov M., Lukić M., Savić S. A 10% lactobionic acid-containing moisturizer reduces skin surface pH without irritation — an in vivo/in vitro study. J Cosmet Dermatol 2019; 18(6): 1705–1710.

Taylor M.B., Yanaki J.S., Draper D.O. et al. Successful short-term and long-term treatment of melasma and postinflammatory hyperpigmentation using vitamin C with a full-face iontophoresis mask and a mandelic/malic acid skin care regimen. J Drugs Dermatol 2013; 12(1): 45–50.

Törmä H. Regulation of keratin expression by retinoids. Dermatoendocrinol 2011; 3(3): 136–140.

Trojahn C., Dobos G., Blume-Peytavi U. et al. The skin barrier function: differences between intrinsic and extrinsic aging. G Ital Dermatol Venereol 2015; 150(6): 687–692.

Truchuelo M., Cerdá P., Fernández L.F. Chemical peeling: a useful tool in the office. Actas Dermosifiliogr 2017; 108(4): 315–322.

VanBuren C.A., Everts H.B. Vitamin A in skin and hair: an update. Nutrients 2022; 14(14): 2952.

van den Bogaard E.H.J, van Geel M., van Vlijmen-Willems I.M.J.J. et al. Deficiency of the human cysteine protease inhibitor cystatin M/E causes hypotrichosis and dry skin. Genet Med 2019; 21(7): 1559–1567.

Virtanen M., Gedde-Dahl T., Mörk N.J. et al. Phenotypic/genotypic correlations in patients with epidermolytic hyperkeratosis and the effects of retinoid therapy on keratin expression. Acta Derm Venereol 2001; 81(3): 163–170.

Voegeli R., Doppler S., Joller P. et al. Increased mass levels of certain serine proteases in the stratum corneum in acute eczematous atopic skin. Int J Cosmet Sci 2011; 33(6): 560–565.

Voegeli R., Rawlings A.V., Breternitz M. et al. Increased stratum corneum serine protease activity in acute eczematous atopic skin. Br J Dermatol 2009; 161(1): 70–77.

Wambier C.G., Lee K.C., Soon S.L. et al. Advanced chemical peels: phenol–croton oil peel. J Am Acad Dermatol 2019; 81(2): 327–336.

Weissler J.M., Carney M.J., Carreras Tartak J.A. et al. The evolution of chemical peeling and modern-day applications. Plast Reconstr Surg 2017; 140(5): 920–929.

Yevglevskis M., Bowskill C.R., Chan C.C. et al. A study on the chiral inversion of mandelic acid in humans. Org Biomol Chem 2014; 12(34): 6737–6744.

Yu R.J., Van Scott E.J. Hydroxycarboxylic acids, N-acetylamino sugars, and N-acetylamino acids. Skinmed 2002; 1(2): 117–122; quiz 125–126.

Zanotti G., Berni R. Plasma retinol-binding protein: structure and interactions with retinol, retinoids, and transthyretin. Vitam Horm 2004; 69: 271–295.

Zdrada J., Odrzywołek W., Deda A. et al. A split-face comparative study to evaluate the efficacy of 50% pyruvic acid against a mixture of glycolic and salicylic acids in the treatment of acne vulgaris. J Cosmet Dermatol 2020; 19(9): 2352–2358.

Zeeuwen P.L. Epidermal differentiation: the role of proteases and their inhibitors. Eur J Cell Biol 2004; 83(11–12): 761–773.

Zhang Z., Lukic M., Savic S. et al. Reinforcement of barrier function — skin repair formulations to deliver physiological lipids into skin. Int J Cosmet Sci 2018; 40(5): 494–501.

Zouboulis C.C., Korge B., Akamatsu H. et al. Effects of 13-cis-retinoic acid, all-trans-retinoic acid, and acitretin on the proliferation, lipid synthesis and keratin expression of cultured human sebocytes in vitro. J Invest Dermatol 1991; 96(5): 792–797.

www.ingramcontent.com/pod-product-compliance
Lightning Source LLC
LaVergne TN
LVHW050310040526
837301LV00003B/29